D1476004

Inspecting Surgical Instruments:
An Illustrated Guide

Rick Schultz

Reviewers

Alex Vrancich

General Manager

Spectrum Surgical Instruments Corp.

Stow, Ohio

Matt Rudolph

Senior Sales Executive

Spectrum Surgical Instruments Corp.

Stow, Ohio

Richard Schule, BS, CST, CRCST, CHMMC, FCS

Manager, Surgical Processing

The Cleveland Clinic Foundation

Cleveland, Ohio

David Narrance, RN, BSN

Nurse Manager and Specialty Clinician, Sterile Processing

MedCentral Health Systems

Mansfield, Ohio

Forward

The surgical instrument represents a significant dollar investment to our customers yet the least amount of time and money is dedicated toward preventive maintenance and continued education for the care and handling of these important medical devices. Surgical instruments having evolved over time are far more sophisticated, intricate, and precise working tools used by the surgeon, nurse, surgical technologist, veterinarian, and other allied health professionals. The vision for this book was clear; create a "one stop shop" for quick refined instrument information.

Mr. Schultz has designed and written this text as a reflection of his vision and passion for education for the care and handling, identification and inspection of surgical instruments. A number of educational documents and programs are available to the central service technician, but none address surgical instrumentation to the breadth and scope as this text. He has successfully integrated detailed instrument photographs, correct nomenclature, inspection points for quality assembly, post operative care instructions, assembly tips and surgical use. As a surgical technologist, educator, lecturer, and manager, I see many uses for this text. The information covered in this text will supplement teaching curriculums across several allied health professions. For any medical student ready to begin their surgical rotation this text would aid in their understanding of instrument utilization.

Implementing any Quality Management System (QMS) requires diligence, sound resources, and a solid education program. To educate the new professional entering into healthcare or to enhance the knowledge of the seasoned healthcare professional handling surgical instruments, I would recommend this text to compliment their on going education efforts. This resource is your "one stop shop" for instrument care and handling.

Richard W. Schule, BS, CST, CRCST, CHMMC, FCS
Manager, Surgical Processing
The Cleveland Clinic, Cleveland Ohio

Introduction

The purpose of this book is to identify inspection points on surgical instruments for both processing and clinical personnel. In addition, points of inspection, sharpness standards, proper names, jaw definitions, lengths, surgical uses, and tray assembly tips are provided along with illustrations. The need for this consolidated information comes from hundreds of lectures I have given throughout the United States and Canada. Proper inspection and testing of surgical instruments provides a quality improvement which benefits the patient and surgeon, as well as an economic gain for the Healthcare Institution.

Executing a surgical procedure takes a lot of teamwork and knowledge. This illustrated guide completes the circle of knowledge and places in the hands of a surgeon an instrument that has been properly inspected.

Acknowledgement

I would like to thank all the Healthcare Professionals that have attended my lectures and in-services. All of your questions and concerns over the years have made it possible for me to formulate this book.

To the employees of Spectrum Surgical: I want to thank each and every one of you for your help, support, and industry knowledge you have developed while serving the fine customers of Spectrum Surgical.

Alex Vrancich, thank you for keeping this project on task and on time, and for sharing your valuable instrument expertise.

As the son of two teachers, I would like to thank my parents for many things, but especially for giving me the ability to teach.

Finally, I would like to thank my family: To Michelle, Patrick, and Scott, who on many vacations saw Dad working on this project. The three of you are the center of my world and I am very proud of you.

The Surgical Instrument Manufacturing Process

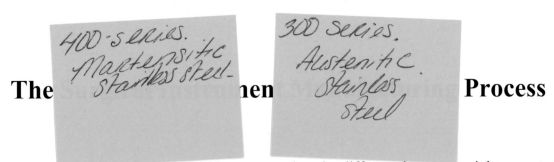

The manufacturing of surgical instruments is quite different than most might expect. In this day of technological advancements, one tends to imagine that instruments are quickly stamped out on an assembly line and are shipped to the customer. However, this is far from the actual process, as the manufacture of surgical instruments demands time consuming hands-on labor from highly skilled craftsmen.

To examine the manufacturing process further, we must begin with the raw materials used to create surgical instruments. Most surgical instruments are produced from stainless steel, however, other materials like titanium, copper and silver are also widely used. Let's begin our discussion by examining stainless steel in more detail.

As there are many types of surgical instruments, there are also several types of stainless steel used in producing surgical instruments. When producing sharp cutting edges, it is appropriate to use a hard steel such as 400 series stainless steel. Instruments produced using 400 series steel include: scissors, osteotomes, chisels, rongeurs, forceps, hemostats, and needle holders. This hardened steel is known as Martensitic stainless steel. The second most popular steel used is 300 series stainless steel, which offers high corrosion resistance, but doesn't offer the hardness properties of 400 series, making it more workable and malleable. Instruments produced using 300 series stainless steel included retractors, cannulas, rib-spreaders, and suction devices, to name a few. This softer type of steel is referred to as Austenitic stainless steel. Titanium is also used to produce lightweight instruments that are extremely corrosion resistant and non-magnetic. Silver and copper are used because of their malleable properties. Instruments made of these substances include trachea tubes and lacrymal probes.

As mentioned, the most common raw material used to produce surgical instruments is stainless steel. This is how it is known in the industry and this is how we will refer to it. However, it is important to note that stainless steel does stain, it does spot and it does rust. It is more appropriate to say that stainless steel is stain resistant, not stain "less". Proper care will ensure that an instrument performs and lasts a long time.

From the stainless steel raw material, we begin to create the instrument. The first step is to develop the forging. The forging is a stamp of the rough outline of an instrument and is made from a heated bar of stainless steel. The heating and cooling process during the creation of an instrument is very important, but one fact remains, a good forging will produce a good instrument. Most high quality forgings come from mills in Germany, but forgings also come from Japan, Pakistan, France and Sweden.

After the creation of the forging, the next step is to grind and mill the forging. First, the excess steel surrounding the forging, known as the flash, is removed. For ring handled instruments, such as scissors and hemostats, more than twenty milling operations will be performed, including the creation of the male and female halves, the cutting of precise serrations, and the machining of the ratchets.

In today's instrument manufacturing environment, there is more reliance on machines, as craftsmen have presses, lathes, CNC milling machines, and drop hammers at their disposal. In years past, an instrument maker would have only a file, a grindstone, and other hand tools. Despite these technical advances, surgical instrument makers must possess a high degree of manual skill. The instrument makers undergo several years of training in the form of an apprenticeship, whereby they train under the guidance of trained and experienced craftsperson. The instrument makers perform hundreds of quality checks and finishing applications to each and every instrument, ensuring the quality of the instrument.

At the completion of the assembly process, instruments undergo a final heating procedure. The instruments are heated to roughly 1500 degrees Fahrenheit (higher or lower depending on the style of instrument), and then are cooled in a controlled fashion. This is what provides the instrument with its hardness. As mentioned before, if this process is not completely controlled, it will result in possible breakage, even under conditions of normal use. For instance, improper heating and cooling could lead to a brittle instrument that breaks easily while performing its normal function. Now that the instruments have been tempered, thus ensuring hardness, we must now improve their resistance to corrosion.

To achieve this, instruments undergo the following processes: polishing and passivation. Polishing is necessary to achieve the instrument's smooth finish, and ultimately determines the final appearance or finish of the instrument. Surgical instruments can be shiny which is called mirror-finish, or can be matte or satin finish, which is a gray colored surface that doesn't reflect light. Both finishes are widely accepted and both create a smooth surface, however, because the mirror finish is smoother, it tends to stain less frequently. Secondly, the instruments undergo a chemical process known as passivation. Passivation uses nitric acid to remove all the iron content still found on the outside layer of the instrument. The removal of this iron helps to build a protective outside layer of chromium oxide. This layer is highly resistant to corrosion and continues to build up throughout the life of the instrument.

The instrument is now ready for final inspection. During final inspection, the instruments will be scrutinized at every turn. Ratchets, tips, scissor blades, serrations, box locks, and spot welds, all will be tested. Finally, the instrument is ready to be etched and packaged. Etching is an acid-based chemical procedure that employs stencils that apply the company name, the part number and the country of origin. Laser etching and stamping are additional methods used for marking instruments.

There you have the surgical instrument manufacturing process. It is a lengthy, detailed endeavor and requires a tremendous amount of experience, skill and craftsmanship. A typical manufacturing cycle from forging to finished instrument usually takes up to six weeks.

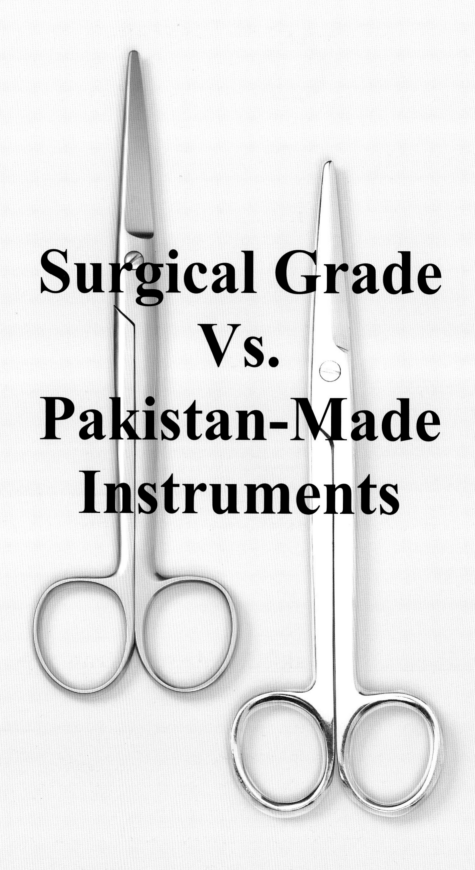

Surgical Grade
Vs.
Pakistan-Made
Instruments

Surgical Grade Instruments

Most instrument sets are comprised of high quality surgical grade instruments. These expensive instruments have many advantages over low-cost Pakistan-made instruments. Although most surgical grade instruments are made in Germany using German stainless steel, some are now manufactured in Malaysia, Hungary, Poland, and Pakistan.

Facts about Surgical Grade Instruments

- Most Surgical Grade instruments are now produced with a matte or satin finish
- Instruments are marked with company name, item number, and country of origin, usually Germany Stainless
- Surgical Grade instruments are almost always backed by a lifetime warranty, which covers manufacturer defects including cracks and rusting
- If properly cared for, surgical grade instruments should last for many years

Pakistan-Made Instruments

Learning to identify and control the use of Pakistan-made instruments is very critical. Pakistan instruments are manufactured to be <u>disposable</u> or <u>semi-disposable.</u> Keeping this in mind, you will find that this is not a low cost alternative to purchasing German-made instruments.

Facts about Pakistan-Made Instruments

- The majority of Pakistan-made instruments have a shiny finish
- To identify, read the marking/etching on the instruments (i.e., Stainless Pakistan)
- You can sterilize Pakistan-made instruments along with German-made instruments; however, the Pakistan-made instrument will rust quickly, which will result in the staining of your German-made instruments
- Never sharpen or repair Pakistan-made instruments because it costs less to buy a new one
- Pakistan-made instruments using Pakistan-made stainless steel rusts very quickly

Metals and Terminology Used In Manufacturing of Surgical Instruments

AISI – American Iron and Steel Institute has identified various stainless steel formulas and classified them.

ASTM – American Society of Testing and Materials sets the standard for metal material.

Austenitic – A stainless steel that cannot be heat-hardened. Stainless steel that falls into this category is 300 series stainless steel, which is highly corrosion resistant.

Martensitic – A stainless steel that can be heat hardened. Stainless steel that falls into this category is 400 series, which is subject to corrosion due to lack of nickel.

Rockwell Scale – A method and scale used to measure the hardness of metals.

Stainless Steel – The most popularly used metal in the manufacturing of surgical instruments. Stainless steel stains and stainless steel rusts.

304 Stainless – Used to make bowls and basins.

316 LVM Stainless – Used to make implantable devices such as pins, plates and screws.

420 Stainless – Pakistan-made and disposable quality instruments are made of this type of stainless steel.

Sterling Silver – Used to make probes and tracheostomy tubes.

Titanium – Very strong and non-magnetic, lightweight metal used for microsurgical instruments. This metal is identified by its blue color and is stronger and lighter than stainless steel.

Tungsten Carbide – An extremely hard metal used in jaws of needleholders and blades of scissors. When tungsten carbide is used, the handle of the instrument will be gold in color.

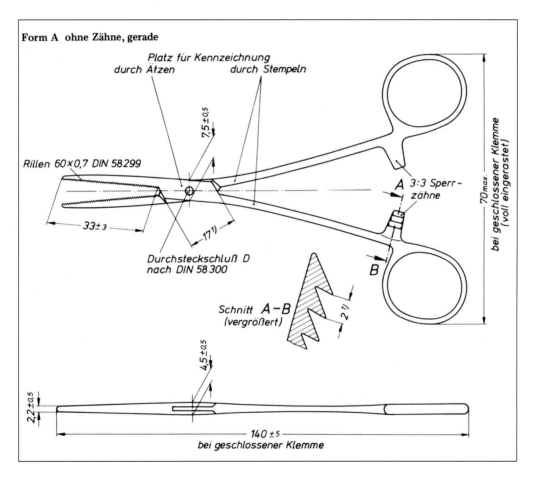

Sample of a German Technical Drawing

Instrument Care
And
Handling

New Instruments

Most professionals will recognize that new instruments feel different. New instruments, especially scissors, feel flawless, and ratcheted instruments can feel stiff. These instruments can feel harder and stiffer because as instruments age, they soften with use and processing. With proper care and use, these devices can last a lifetime. It's important to realize, however, that even the highest-grade instruments will initially feel harder and will stain. New instruments tend to be more magnetic in the box locks, serrations, and ratchets due to the manufacturing process transferring the magnetism. This magnetism gradually wears off and this is one of the reasons newer instruments tend to stain more rapidly.

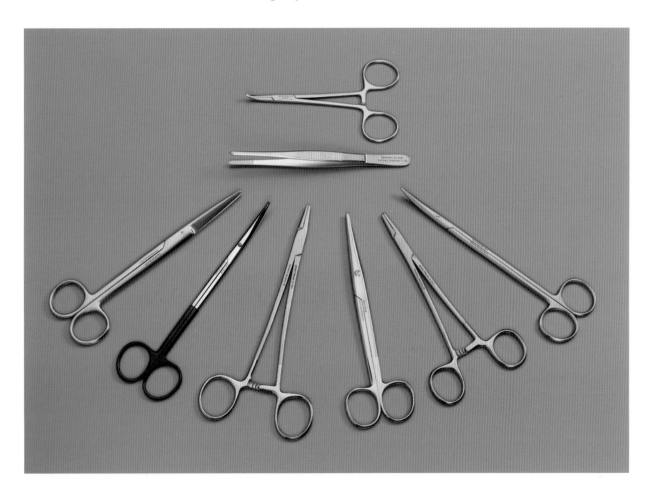

Enemies of Surgical Instruments

- Allowing blood to dry onto instruments

- Soaking instruments in water

- Soaking instruments in saline

- Any and all long-term soaking will damage surgical instruments

- Sterilizing instruments with ratchets closed

- Improper use of the instrument

- Rough handling/dumping of instruments

- The use of improper cleaning solutions and lubricants

- Allowing water to dry onto instruments

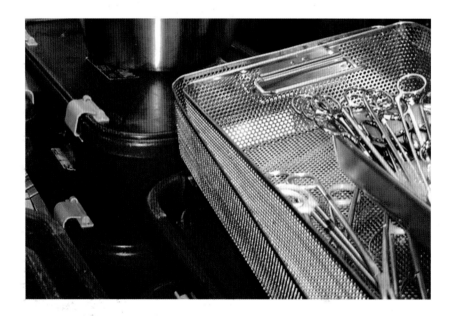

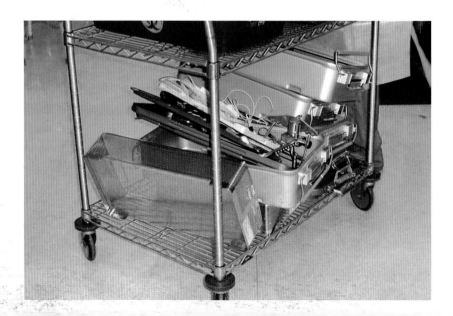

Post Operative Care of Surgical Instruments

Never allow blood to dry onto surgical instruments. Immediately (within 10-20 minutes) after the case, separate the rings of the instruments and begin the decontamination process (as seen in the top photo below). To prevent blood from drying onto instruments, simply saturate a towel with tap water and lay over the bloody, contaminated instruments (see the bottom photo below). The use of spray-on moisturizers is also a very effective way to prevent the blood from drying, along with the use of enzymatic solutions.

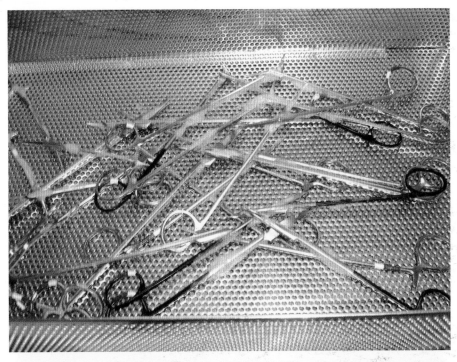

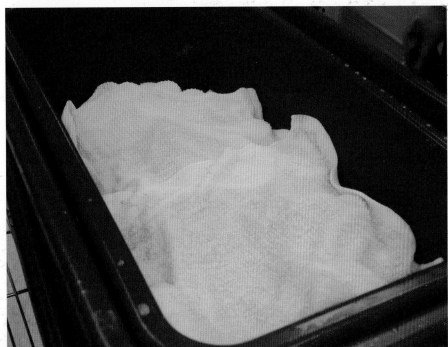

Manual Washing

Manual washing prior to mechanical washing should be kept to a minimum. The most important factor is soap selection, which should be of neutral pH. Never use a soap that is not exclusively designed to be used on surgical instruments. The manual washing step is where brushing occurs to clean box locks, serrations and lumens.

Soaps to avoid are:

- Housekeeping soaps
- Laundry soaps
- Surgeon's hand scrub
- Iodine based soaps

Ultrasonic Cleaning

The cleaning of surgical instruments with ultrasonic energy is the single best practice you can do. This technology removes bioburden very efficiently and is very safe for instruments. The longer the instruments are in the ultrasonic cleaner, the cleaner the instruments will be. Only use a neutral pH ultrasonic solution and never put manual instrument soap in the ultrasonic cleaner.

Other Facts:

- Temperature of tank solution can improve performance with heated solution
- Change solution daily or when bioburden is noticed in tank
- The longer instruments are left in, the better
- Do not overload ultrasonic cleaner as this reduces its cleaning efficiency
- Instruments should always be in the open position when placed in the ultrasonic cleaner

Rinsing of Instruments

After manual washing or ultrasonic cleaning, rinse the surgical instruments with water, preferably with distilled water. Remove residue left on from detergents, both from ultrasonic and machine washing.

Drying of Instruments

Never allow water to dry onto surgical instruments as this will result in water spots, which will turn into stains.

Lubrication

All hinged surgical instruments need lubrication after each use. A spray-on lubricant or machine applied lubrication works best. Neutral pH lubricants are recommended. Mineral based lubricants should never be used as steam cannot penetrate mineral oils, and instruments will not achieve sterility.

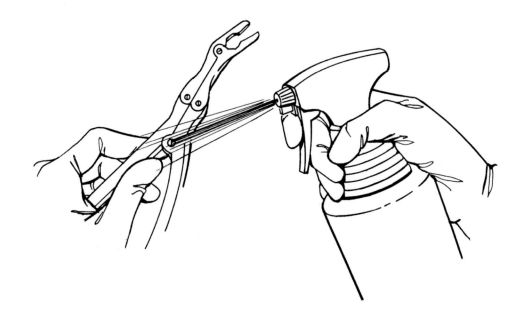

How to Determine If an Instrument
Is Rusted *or* Stained

Stains can be removed whereas rust will leave permanent (pitting) damage on instruments. To determine if a brown/orange discoloration is a stain or rust, use the eraser test. Simply rub a pencil eraser over the discoloration. If the discoloration is removed and the surface metal underneath is smooth and clean, this is a stain. However, if the discoloration is removed with the pencil eraser and a pit mark appears under the discoloration, this is corrosion, which will continually rust.

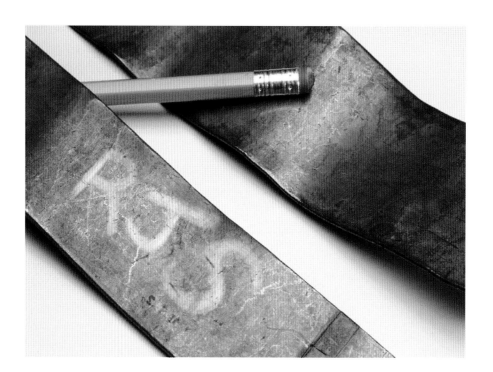

Troubleshooting Stain Guide

Brown/Orange Stains – Most brown/orange stains are not rust. This stain color is a result of high pH surface deposits caused by any of the following: chlorhexidine usage, improper soaps and detergents, cold sterilization solution, possibly baked-on blood, soaking in saline, or using laundry soap.

Dark Brown/Black Stains – Low pH (less than 6) acid stain. May be caused by improper detergents and soaps and/or dried blood.

Bluish Black Stains – Reverse plating may occur when different metals are ultrasonically processed together. For example, stainless steel instruments processed with chrome instruments will cause a stain color reaction. Exposure to saline, blood, or potassium chloride will cause this bluish black stain to occur.

Multicolor Stains – Excessive heat by a localized "hot spot" in the processing cycle.

Light and Dark Spots – Water spots from allowing instruments to air-dry. With slow evaporation, the minerals (sodium, calcium, and magnesium) are left on the instrument's surface.

Bluish Gray Stains – Cold sterilization solution being used outside manufacturer guidelines.

Black Stains – Possible exposure to ammonia.

The Use of Saline

The soaking and rinsing of stainless steel instruments with saline will destroy the instruments. The majority of surgical instrument manufacturers state in their warranties, "the soaking/use of saline will void the warranty." Clinically use saline as directed, however, eliminate any and all contact with saline in the instrument cleaning process.

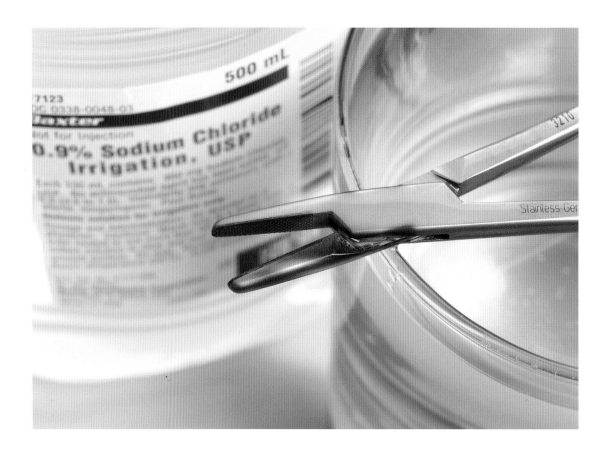

The Care of Bariatric Instruments

The care, handling, and inspection of Bariatric Instruments are exactly the same as with standard instruments. Key points of inspection include the box lock area and the jaws. The only significant difference pertaining to Bariatric Instruments is the overall length of the instruments.

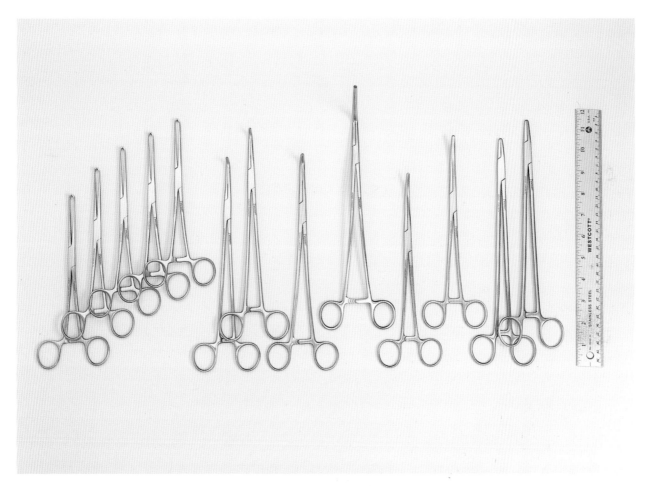

Bariatric Instruments

Instrument Stringers

Instrument Stringers allow for:

- Safer handling of instruments
- Faster set-up of sterile field
- Ratchets to stay open during sterilization
- More efficient organization of the tray assembly process

Instrument Stringers are produced in various widths and lengths. The most common width is 2.5 inches with the most common length being 10 inches. After selecting size, there are various stringer closure systems to choose from.

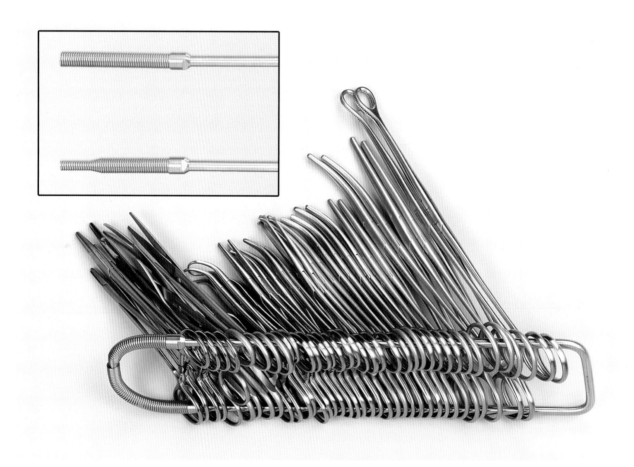

Quick Rack Stringer

Repair Tags

The use of repair tags facilitates precise communication between the operating room and the sterile processing department. Placing 3-5 new repair tags in each set prior to sterilization allows the tags to be available on the sterile field. Once a dull or damaged instrument is discovered during the procedure, a sterile repair tag can then be placed on the instrument. This system precisely identifies the defective instrument and prevents unnecessary repairs.

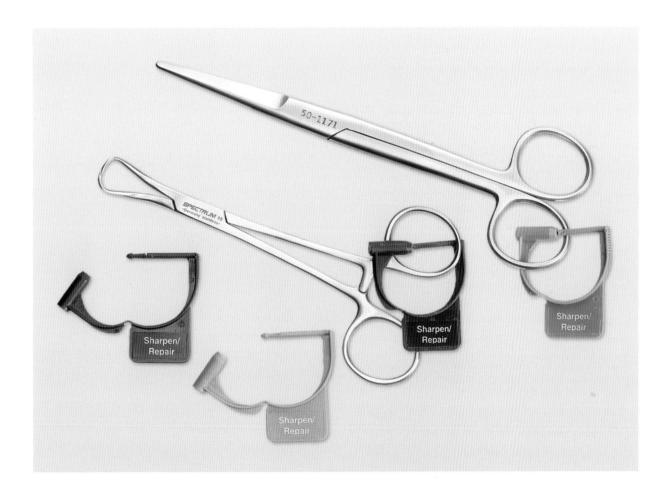

Tip Protectors

The use of Tip Protectors is a good practice that protects valuable instruments and scopes from being damaged. Many times the damage to an instrument from not using Tip Protectors is not repairable, thus making it necessary to replace the instrument. Tip Protectors are manufactured both vented (with holes) and non-vented (without holes). Vented Tip Protectors are safer to use due to the fact that they are easier to remove from the instrument, which reduces possible finger punctures. The other advantage of the vented Tip Protector is the improved exposure of the sterilant to the device surface.

Places to use Tip Protectors:

- Tips of pointed scissors
- Tips of sharp instruments
- Skin hooks
- Distal tip of rigid scopes
- Cutting edges of osteotomes

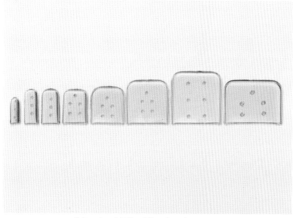

Vented Tip Protectors

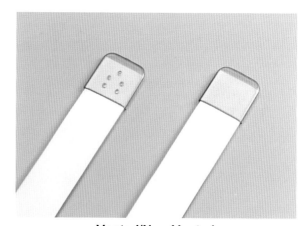

Vented/Non-Vented

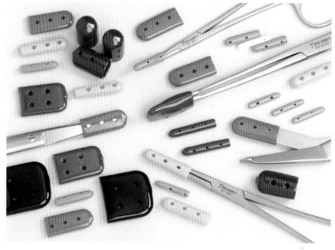

Metal Instrument Protection Cases

The use of metal storage/sterilization cases for specific instruments has several valuable benefits:

- Keeps high demand instruments organized
- Reduces the opportunity for misplacing a certain sized instrument
- Protects the cutting edges of the instruments
- Reduces the number of times the instruments have to be sharpened
- Presents very efficiently and in an organized fashion in the sterile field

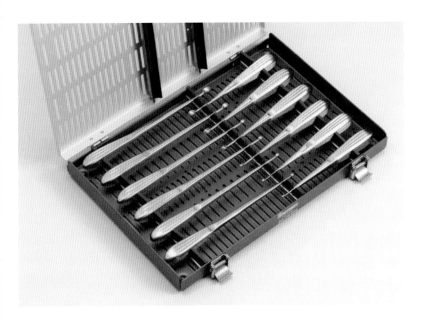

Curette Rack

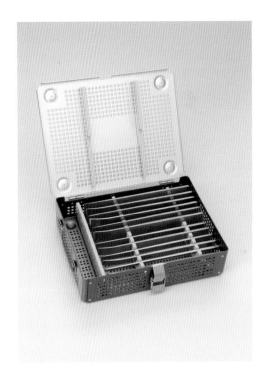

Lambotte Osteotome Rack

Instrument Marking Tape Application

Instructions

1) Clean fingers with alcohol to remove oils, grease, and dirt.

2) Wipe tape site with alcohol to remove any lubricant.

3) Tape length should be only 1 – 1 1/2 times around and applied with firm tension.

4) After tape is applied, autoclave instruments. The heat will assist with the bonding of the tape.

5) Tape the shanks of all instruments. Avoid instrument rings. Wrapping tape 1 – 1 1/2 times around will not interfere with the closing of most scissor tips.

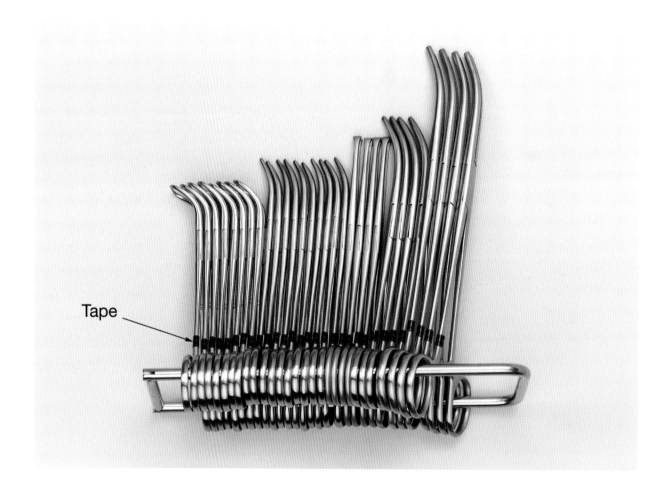

Tape

Cleaning Brushes

For as long as surgical instruments have been used, cleaning brushes have been used to help with the decontamination process. Once while reviewing a book about American-Made surgical instruments, I noticed that a Civil War amputation set had its own cleaning brush in the set. No longer do we use industrial brushes, toothbrushes, or even surgeon's hand scrub brushes to do our cleaning. Instead we have brushes for all cleaning purposes. Cleaning brushes are now made for cleaning the smallest hand held instruments in addition to suction tubes, laparoscopic instruments, and flexible endoscopes.

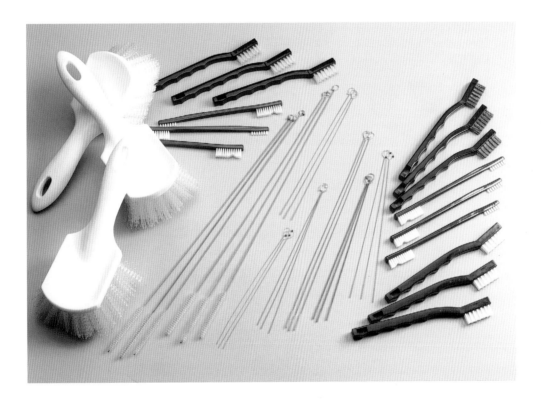

The manufacturing of cleaning brushes has also come a long way in the past few years. Many brushes are known as wire twisted (see photo below), whereby two strands of wire are twisted together to hold the nylon bristles in place. In years past, this wire was often made of galvanized steel, which easily rusted and limited the life of the brush. Today most brushes are made using only medical grade nylon with surgical stainless steel wire. The latest improvement in brush technology is the use of antimicrobial nylon bristles, which combined with stainless steel wire, extends the life of the brush. Please look now to the photo below, which shows a small brush being put through a Frazier suction tube.

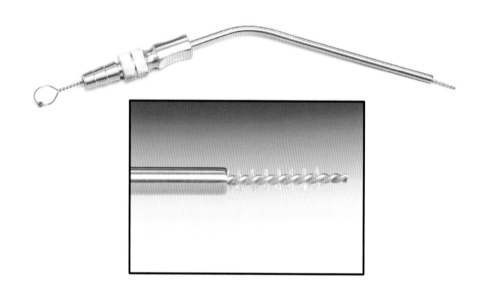

As mentioned previously, there are brushes for cleaning almost everything, and it is important to use the appropriate brush. For instance, if you use a brush with a diameter that is too large, the brush does not effectively clean. If the bristle diameter is too small, the brush will not touch the sides of the lumen and will not clean. The photo below is of a Yankauer suction tube, and you will notice a larger diameter brush being used than in the previous photo.

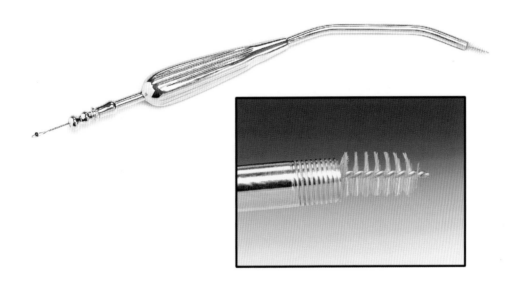

IMPORTANT FACT: When brushing, it is important that all bristles exit the distal tip of the instrument being cleaned (see diagram below). If we fail to use a brush long enough to exit completely, we will simply push the dirt to the spot where we stop. So remember, when brushing, the brush must always exit completely.

The ability to clean an instrument is now the main consideration when producing surgical instruments, and many changes have occurred. These changes have made instruments easier to assemble and disassemble, which makes them more cleanable. Two examples include laparoscopic instrumentation and Kerrison Laminectomy Rongeurs. Laparoscopic instruments have been used for years, but during that time production techniques have changed that now allow Lap instruments to be completely disassembled. Once the instrument is disassembled, it can be cleaned using a cleaning brush (see photos below).

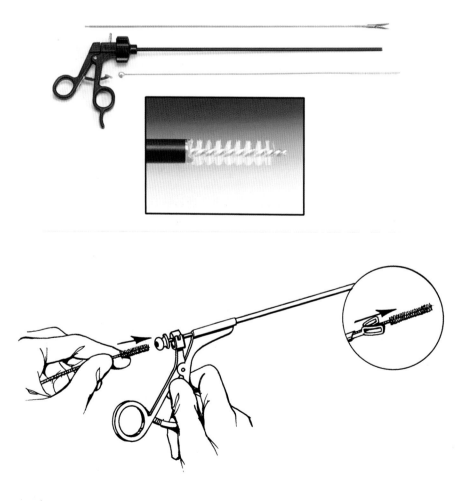

Stainless Steel Cleaning Brushes

In addition to the wire twisted brushes shown in the previous images, there are several other styles of brushes. The most popular is the toothbrush style brushes, shown in the photo below. These brushes are available in brass, nylon, and stainless steel. It is recommended that brass bristles not be used, as mixing metals is not recommended (Much the same as in ultrasonic cleaning). Nylon bristle brushes are great for cleaning general instruments, such as hemostats, needle holders, and retractors. The bristles are safe and stiff enough to help with most cleaning applications. However, sometimes a more aggressive cleaning brush is required. This is especially true when cleaning serrations and box locks of hemostats, DeBakey forceps, needleholder jaws, and other hard-to-clean areas. The ideal brush for these situations is the stainless steel bristle brush.

There are many opponents of the stainless steel instrument cleaning brush. They claim that the stainless steel bristles harm instruments because they scratch the surface of stainless steel instruments. This is not the case. When examining the photo below, you will notice two stainless steel bristled brushes. The brush on the left has been used extensively to clean instruments; the one on the right has never been used. This comparison shows us that the bristles do not remain intact during the cleaning process, they give way and bend, and therefore do not harm the instruments they are cleaning. A recent study shows through Scanning Electron Microscope (SEM) technology that no harm is caused by the stainless steel bristles, making them the perfect brush for hard-to-clean debris. However, the stainless steel cleaning brush should never be used on insulated or coated instruments. Examples include insulated laparoscopic instruments, bipolar forceps, coated electrosurgical instruments, and ebonized laser-finished instruments. The brush will damage these protective coatings and should never be used in these situations.

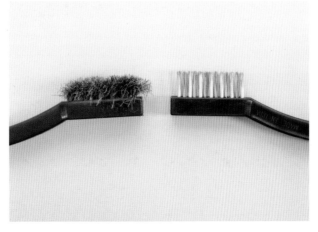

Surgical Instrument Repair

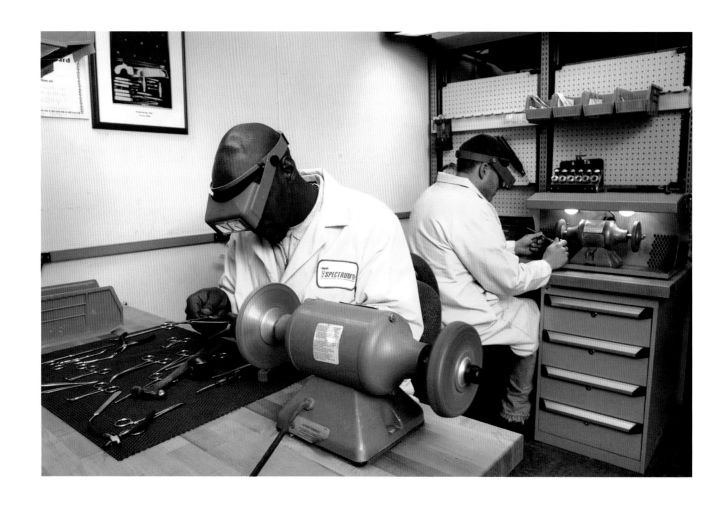

Evaluating a Repair Vendor

The art of surgical instrument restoration is not something that can be learned overnight. Much like the instrument makers in Germany, it takes years for a repair technician to develop the skills necessary for such delicate and precise work. In today's healthcare market, instrument repair is on the rise as facilities strive to protect and maintain their million-dollar surgical instrument inventories. It has been proven that it is cost effective to maintain surgical instruments in lieu of purchasing new equipment. The scores of factors surrounding the selection of a repair vendor make this a most difficult decision, and not making the right choice could end up costing your facility time, money, and needless aggravation. The following questions will help you put your surgical instrument repair vendor to the test.

1) What is the vendor's availability?
2) Is your repair vendor buffing off catalogue numbers?
3) Is your repair vendor repairing Pakistan-made instruments?
4) Is your repair vendor changing the finish of your instruments?
5) Does your repair vendor replace needle holder jaws on-location?
6) Does your repair vendor send only one technician?
7) Does your repair vendor offer instrument tracking and quality assurance programs?
8) Does your repair vendor return broken or non-repairable instruments?
9) Does your repair vendor provide educational services?
10) Is your instrument vendor able to service specialty instruments?
11) Does your repair vendor inspect and service your instrument board?
12) Have you toured your mobile repair laboratory?
13) Does your vendor offer a full range of repair capabilities?

A good strategy to employ during the selection process is to schedule trial service days with all prospective vendors. A good repair company will be more than willing to showcase their capabilities and try to earn your business. During this trial it is important that you execute the strategies discussed above and make your decision based on the value you receive and the level of service provided.

Secondly, never underestimate the value that a repair vendor can provide through education. A vendor that helps your efforts and serves as a consultant by making suggestions for improvement will certainly save you money over the long term. Choosing the right vendor is one of the best decisions you will make, as it will save your budget, save your time and, most importantly, save you from needless stress and aggravation.

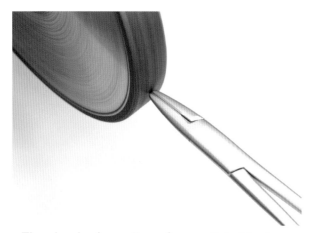

The shaping/rounding of a needleholder jaw

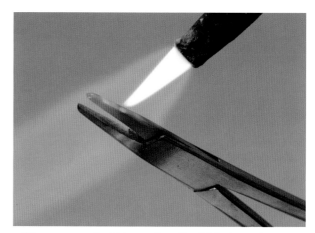

The removal of Tungsten Carbide Inserts

What to Expect From a Repair Vendor

1) **Availability:** A repair vendor should be available seven days a week. The most frequently used sets are usually only available to be serviced on evenings or weekends.

2) **Buffing Off Catalog Numbers**: See page 41

3) **Pakistan-Made Instruments:** See page 5

4) **Changing the Finish:** German-made instruments are produced in two colors; matte finish (gray) and mirror finish (shiny). Matte finish is non-reflective and does not produce glare and mirror finish is a smoother finish, which will resist staining. Instruments sent out for repair should be restored without altering the finish.

5) **Needleholders:** Should only be repaired on location.

6) **One Technician:** The more technicians the better, and the more value-added services you receive.

7) **Instrument Tracking:** The repair vendor should provide this service for the hospital.

8) **Broken Instruments:** All instruments should be returned to the hospital for warranty usage.

9) **Education:** Accredited educational programs should be provided yearly by your vendor.

10) **Specialty Instruments:** Yes, besides sharpening services, all complex specialty instruments should be serviced on location.

11) **Instrument Board:** The back-up instruments are as important to be serviced as the sets.

12) **Tour Repair Vehicles:** Visit the repair vehicle to determine if it is a professional repair vehicle providing professional services.

13) **Full Range:** Besides servicing surgical instruments, a cost effective vendor will service scopes, power equipment, and electrical surgical instruments.

Sharpness Testing Standards

Test Standard for General Scissors Larger than 4.5"

Using red test material, 3/4 of the scissor blade should cut completely through test material three times without snagging, especially at the tip. The cutting action should be smooth when opening and closing scissors.

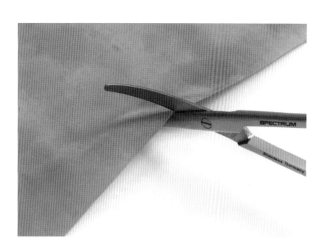 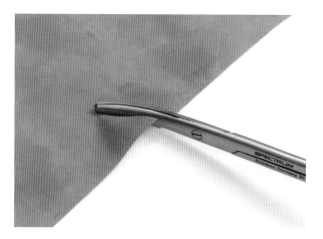

Test Standard for Micro Scissors Smaller than 4.5"

Using yellow test material, 3/4 of the scissor blade should cut completely through test material three times without snagging, especially at the tip. The cutting action should be smooth when opening and closing scissors.

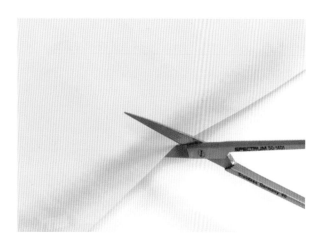 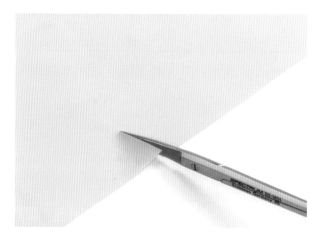

Test Standard for Osteotomes

Never sharpen if overall length is 1.5" less than original specification. A sharpened Osteotome should be 90° at the corners and look like a church steeple from the side. Test for sharpness using a plastic dowel rod at a 45° angle and the Osteotome should bite into the dowel rod. Visual inspection of edge can identify damaged cutting surface.

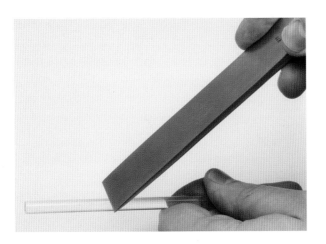 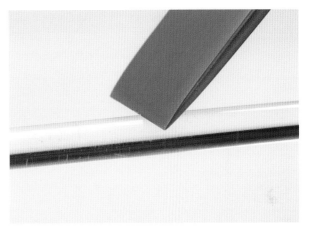

Test Standard for Curettes

Edges are free of nicks and burrs. Test for sharpness using a plastic dowel rod. Curette's sharpened edges should stick into the plastic rod and remove a sample. Visual inspection of edge can identify damaged cutting surface.

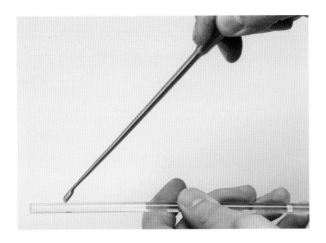 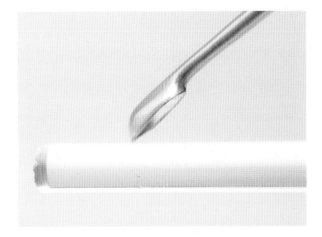

Test Standard for Laparoscopic Scissor

Blades open and close smoothly. Blades will cut through a single layer of facial tissue paper without snagging.

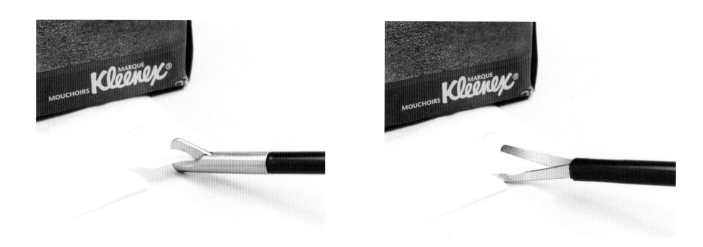

Test Standard for Knives

Blades are free of nicks and when sharpened on both sides will stick to a plastic dowel rod.

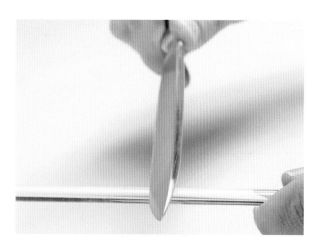 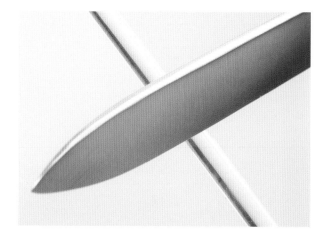

Test Standard for Kerrison Rongeurs

Jaws will cut cleanly through a single layer of an index card without tearing. Rongeur will open and close smoothly and should spring open. Interlocking springs should be free of cracks.

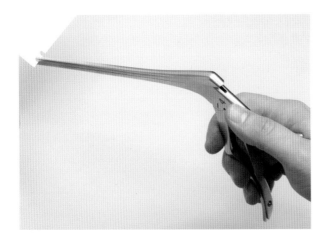
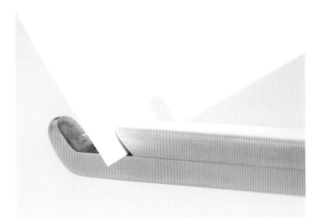

Test Standard for Double Action Rongeurs

Jaws will cut cleanly through a single layer of an index card without tearing. Rongeur will open and close smoothly and should spring open. Interlocking springs should be free of cracks.

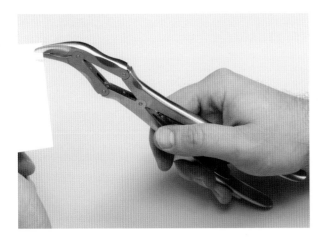
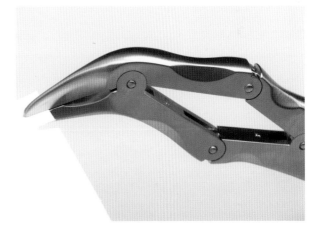

Test Standard for Single Action Rongeurs

Jaws will cut cleanly through a single layer of an index card without tearing. Rongeur will open and close smoothly and should spring open. Interlocking springs should be free of cracks.

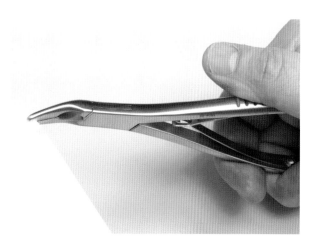 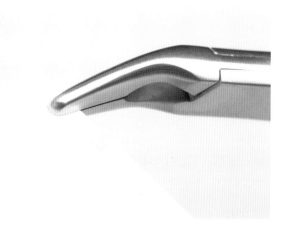

Test Standard for Gouges

Edges are free of nicks and burrs. Test for sharpness using a plastic dowel rod. Edges should stick when holding gouge at a 45° angle. Visually inspect edge for damage to the cutting surface.

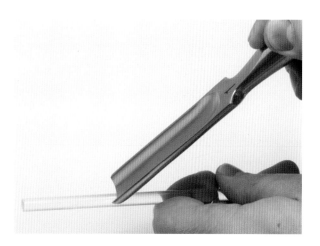 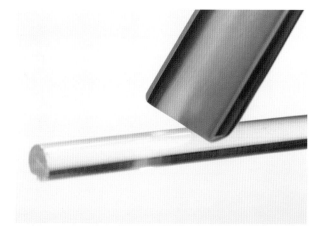

Test Standard for Pituitary Rongeurs

3/4 of jaws should make a firm imprint onto an index card. Inspect imprint for consistency.

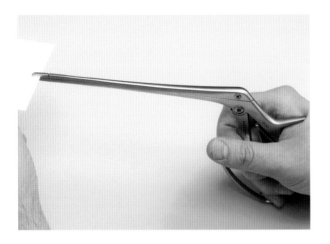 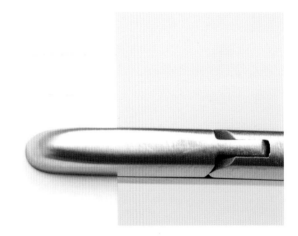

Test Standard for Arthroscopy Punches

This instrument should punch cleanly through a thin piece of leather without tearing or snagging.

Opens and closes smoothly without clicking. This test standard must be OEM approved.

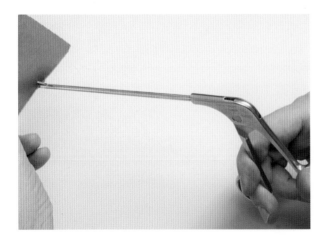 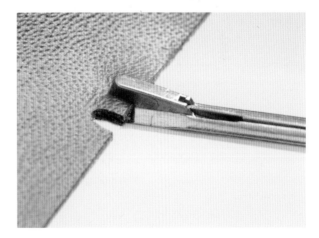

Test Standard for Cervical Biopsy Punches

Should punch cleanly through two layers of facial tissue without snagging or tearing. Springs should be inspected and free of cracks.

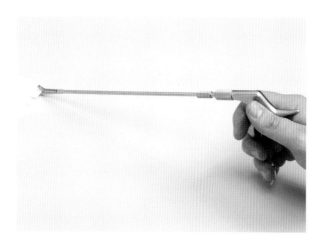 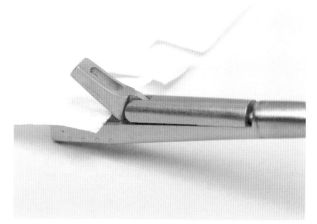

Test Standard for Lister Bandage Scissor

3/4 of the blade's length should cut through a towel without pinching or snagging the towel.

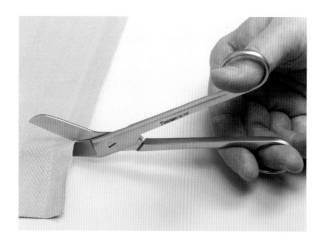 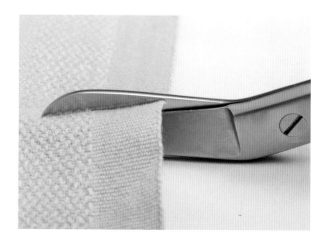

Test Standard for Bone Cutters, Pin Cutters, and Nail Nippers

3/4 of the blade's length should cut completely through an index card.

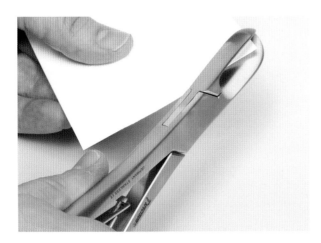 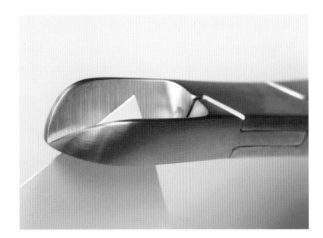

Ratchet Testing; Hemostats and Needleholders

Ratchets will come out of alignment when twisting action is applied. To test a ratchet, engage ratchet on the first click, then softly tap the instrument on a flat surface. If the instruments springs open or simply becomes disengaged, the instrument needs to be repaired.

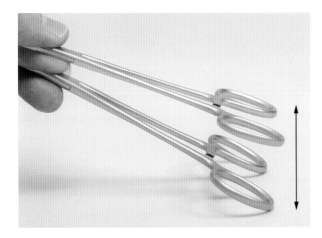 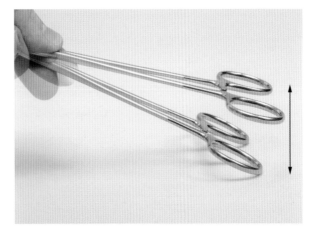

Test Standard for Clipper Blades

Testing twine is inserted into the blades on the far left, middle, and far right of blade. Blades should cut cleanly through the material without snagging or tearing. There should be no broken teeth on either the cutter blade or comb blade.

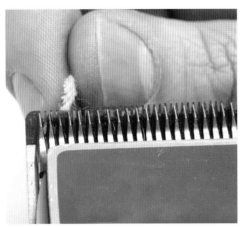 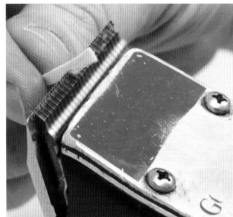 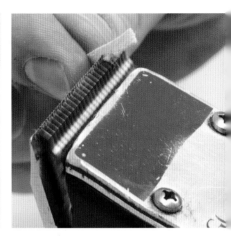

Magnetism

Surgical instruments can become magnetized. The most common cause of this is placing instruments near any electric motor or near magnetic instrument pads or magnetic needle counters. Demagnetization can be performed by your repair vendor or by the hospital's instrument processing staff using a demagnetizer. A demagnetizer can also be purchased from any larger industrial hardware supplier, such as McMaster-Carr. To demagnetize, move instrument slowly over device, this will pull the magnetism out of the instrument.

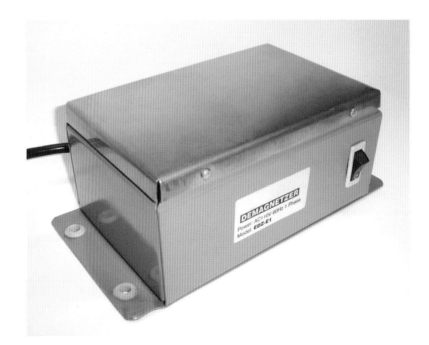

Buffing Off Catalog Numbers in the Repair Lab

The practice of the Repair Vendor buffing/polishing off catalog numbers should be eliminated. The hospital must require the Repair Vendor to protect the catalog numbers because:

1). Buffing the numbers off will void the warranty on the instrument

2). It makes the re-ordering process more difficult

3). It can create litigation issues

4). It can affect the count sheet/tray assembly identification process

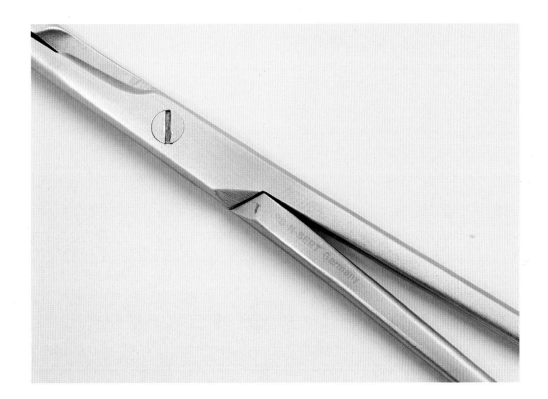

Scissors

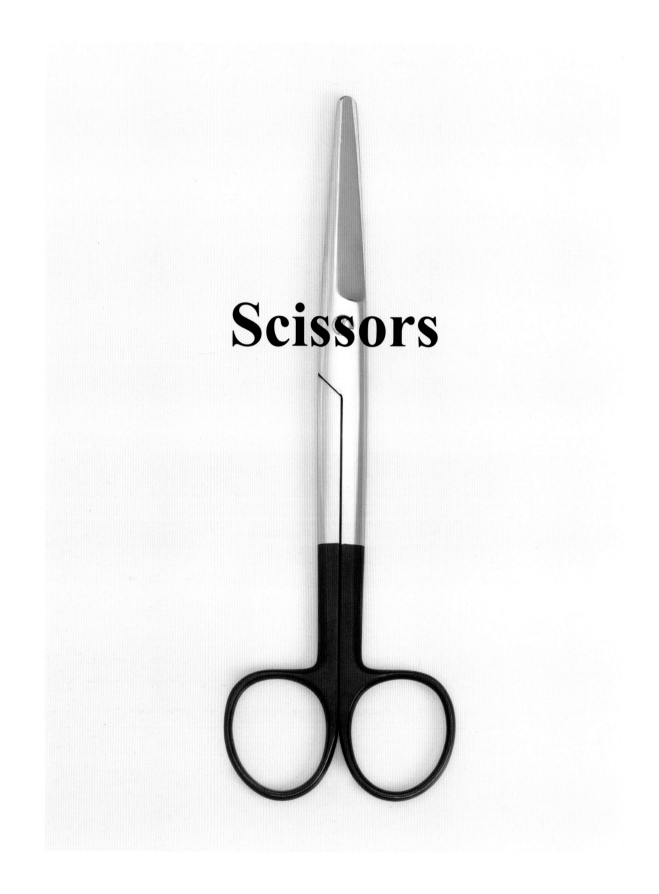

Scissors – Instruments used to cut, incise, and/or dissect tissue.

Facts about Scissors

- All scissors are designed to be re-sharpened
- The feel of scissors should be a smooth slide as you open and close
- Gold handled scissors do stay sharper longer, however, you cannot replace the Tungsten Carbide edges
- Black handled scissors are the sharpest scissors available, however, they go dull the quickest
- Scissors go dull at the distal tip first
- Scissors crack in the screw hinge area
- The weakest part of scissors is the distal tip

Points of Inspection:

- **Blunt Tips:** Scissor tips should be rounded in order to prevent puncturing and tearing. Inspect tips for corrosion and burs.

- **Sharp Tips:** Scissor tips are very fragile, so make sure both tips are present. Inspect sharp tips for bending or damage.

- **Blades:** Inspect blades for chips or burs on cutting surface. If scissor has tungsten carbide blades (gold handles) inspect tungsten carbide insert for cracks. Also, inspect union where tungsten carbide meets the stainless steel for signs of pitting.

- **Screw Hinged Area**: Inspect both sides for the presence of cracking and bioburden trapped in head of the screw. The screw hinge area is most prone to bioburden and staining.

- **Rings:** Inspect the rings for cracks.

- **Scissor Action:** To inspect the cutting action of a scissor, simply open and close the scissor three to four times. This opening and closing action should be a smooth glide as the scissor closes.

- The scissor should not be:
    1. Loose
    2. Tight and grinding
    3. Jumping

The scissor action test is an important inspection next to sharpness testing. The action of a scissor is the surgeon's first impression.

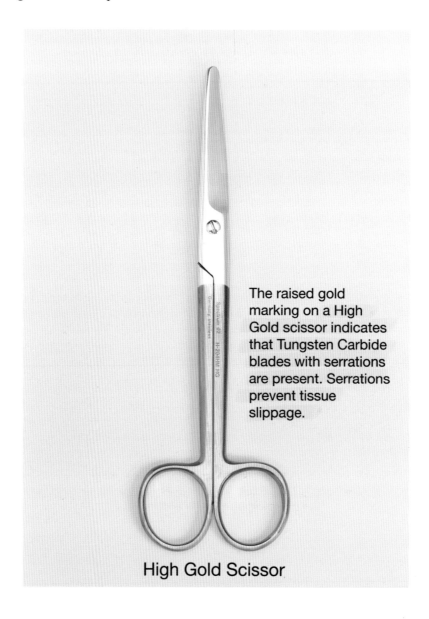

The raised gold marking on a High Gold scissor indicates that Tungsten Carbide blades with serrations are present. Serrations prevent tissue slippage.

High Gold Scissor

Sharpness Testing for Scissors Larger than 4.5"

Test Material: Red scissor test material

     Implementation Plan: Select two to three days per week in which all scissors processed that day will be tested. Issue both test materials and instruct the staff to test the scissors prior to tray assembly. This proactive approach will eventually put only sharp scissors in the surgeon's hand. Caution: material contains latex, however, non-latex materials are now available.

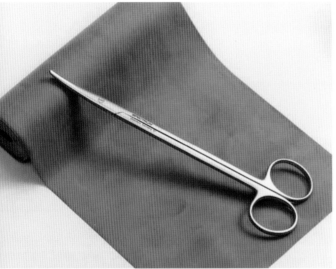

Photo 1: Red test material for scissors larger than 4.5" inches.

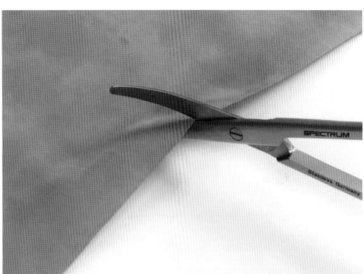

Photo 2: Make two to three cuts making sure scissor cuts all the way through to the tip of scissor. The tips of the scissor are the first area to go dull.

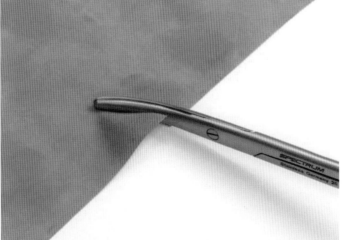

Photo 3: Scissors cut cleanly through to the tip. No snagging or catching indicates that the scissor is surgically sharp.

Sharpness Testing for Scissors Smaller than 4.5"

Test Material: Yellow scissor test material

Implementation Plan: Select two to three days per week in which all scissors processed that day will be tested. Issue both test materials and instruct the staff to test the scissors prior to tray assembly. This proactive approach will eventually put only sharp scissors in the surgeon's hand. Caution: material contains latex, however, non-latex materials are now available.

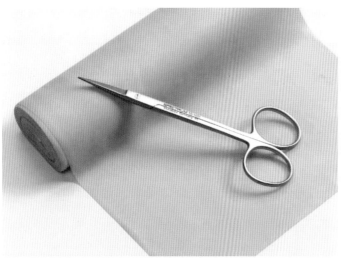

Photo 4: Make two to three cuts making sure scissor cuts all the way through to the tip of scissor. The tips of the scissor are the first area to go dull.

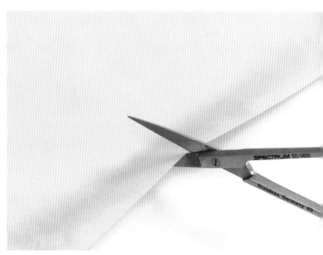

Photo 5: Make two to three cuts making sure scissor cuts all the way through to the tip of scissor. The tips of the scissor are the first area to go dull.

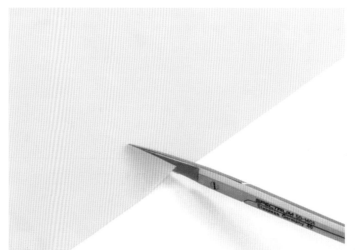

Photo 6: Scissors cut cleanly through to the tip. No snagging or catching indicates that the scissor is surgically sharp.

Scissors

Most surgical scissors are produced with various blade definitions depending on surgical specialty and material being cut. The three different blade definitions are:

Stainless Blades- Scissors with stainless blades are the most common. The entire scissor is made out of the exact same metal (stainless steel) and there are no distinct ring colors.

Tungsten Carbide Blades- Inserted only along the cutting surface of the blade is the metal tungsten carbide. These metal strips are much harder than stainless steel. Once sharpened, these tungsten carbide blades stay sharper longer and are attached to the stainless scissor by welding or vacuum brazing. These tungsten carbide insert strips cannot be replaced once they become sharpened down. Tungsten carbide scissors have gold rings to distinguish this design.

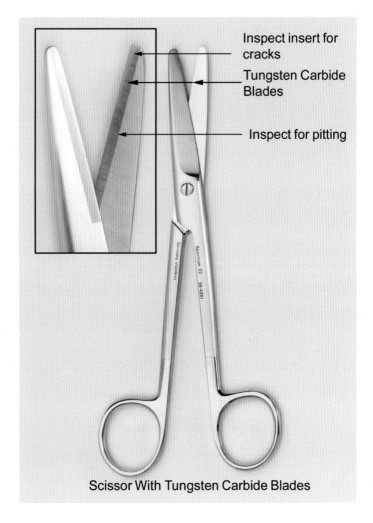

Inspect insert for cracks

Tungsten Carbide Blades

Inspect for pitting

Scissor With Tungsten Carbide Blades

Black Handled Scissors-These scissors are known as Microgrind™ or Supercut™ scissors in the industry. The unique feature of these scissors is the sharpening technique placed on one of the blades. This scissor has a blade that will lance/slice through tissue due to its "knife edge" sharpening technique. All other scissors crush, resulting in cutting, whereas the black handled scissor slices tissue. Black handled scissors require special sharpening techniques and must be resharpened three to four times a year. The unique feature of these scissors is the black colored rings.

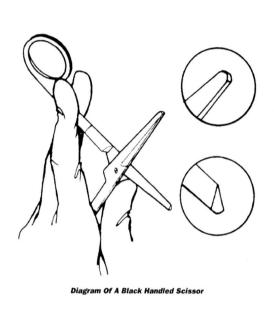

Diagram Of A Black Handled Scissor

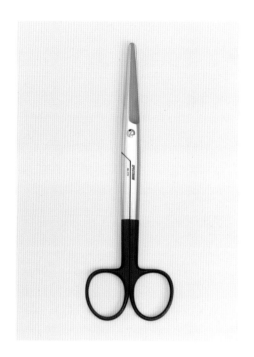

Post-Operative Care: Separate the rings of the scissor completely and never allow blood to dry onto scissors. To prevent blood from drying onto scissors and within twenty minutes of post-op, soak instruments in an enzymatic solution or place a moist towel saturated with water over the scissors.

Scissor Blade Cracking

Gold handled scissors contain cutting blades made of tungsten carbide. Tungsten carbide blades stay sharper longer due to its hardness. Inspect tungsten carbide blades for cracks prior to tray assembly. If a crack is discovered, remove the scissor from the set and send it back to the manufacturer for warranty replacement.

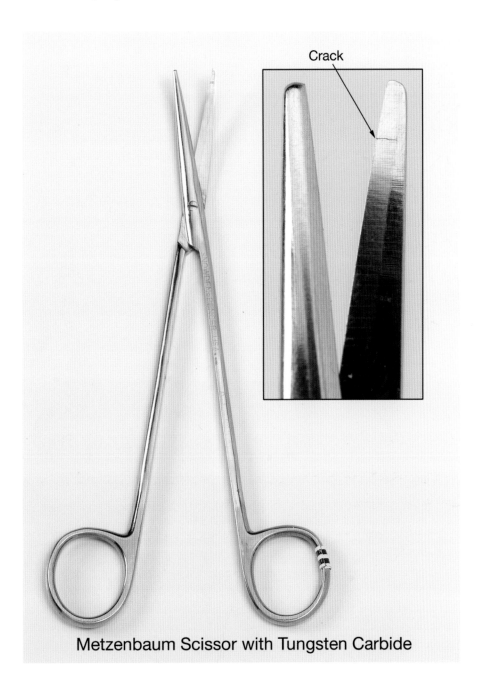

Metzenbaum Scissor with Tungsten Carbide

Mayo Scissor

Proper Name: Mayo Scissor

Other Names: Mayos, Suture Scissors

Similar Instruments with Same Inspections: Mayo Noble, Mayo Sistrunk

Length: 6.75"

Surgical Use: Cutting and dissecting tissue

Tray Assembly Tips: Keep rings slightly separated and tips of scissors going in same direction

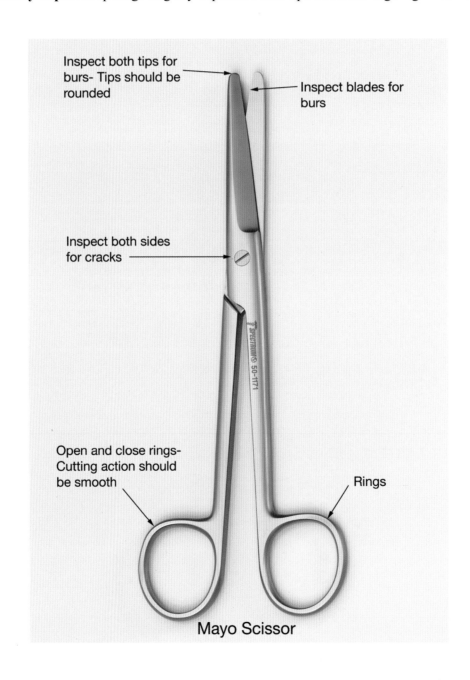

Inspect both tips for burs- Tips should be rounded

Inspect blades for burs

Inspect both sides for cracks

Open and close rings- Cutting action should be smooth

Rings

Mayo Scissor

Metzenbaum Scissor

Proper Name: Metzenbaum Scissor

Other Names: Metz, Nelson, Delicate Scissor, Tissue Scissor

Length: 7"

Surgical Use: For cutting delicate tissue and blunt dissection

Tray Assembly Tips: Keep rings slightly separated and tips of scissors going in same direction

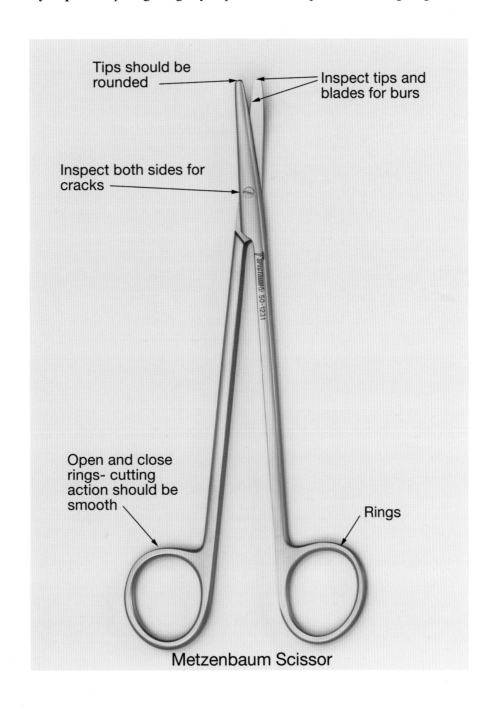

Tips should be rounded

Inspect tips and blades for burs

Inspect both sides for cracks

Open and close rings- cutting action should be smooth

Rings

Metzenbaum Scissor

Sharp/Blunt Operating Scissor

Proper Name: Sharp/Blunt Operating Scissor

Other Names: Sharp/Blunt, Nurse's Scissor, Suture Scissor, O.R. Scissor

Similar Instruments with Same Inspections: Sims

Length: 4.5", 5", 5.5", 6", and 6.5"

Surgical Use: Cutting and dissecting tissue and cutting surgical drapes

Tray Assembly Tips: Keep rings slightly separated and tips of scissors going in same direction

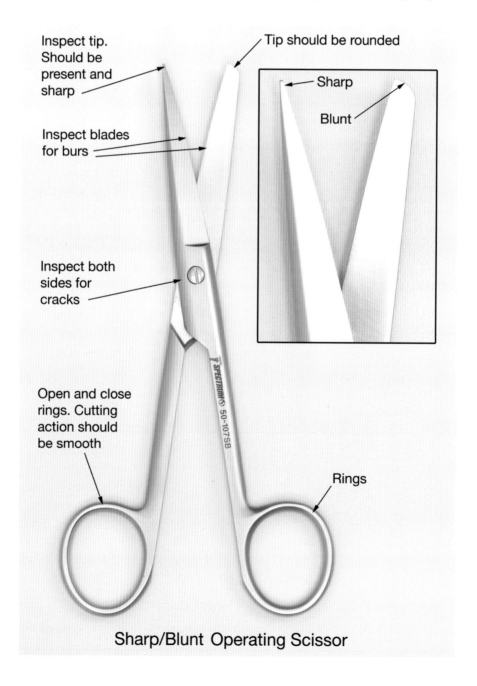

Inspect tip. Should be present and sharp

Tip should be rounded

Sharp

Blunt

Inspect blades for burs

Inspect both sides for cracks

Open and close rings. Cutting action should be smooth

SPECTRUM 50-107SB

Rings

Sharp/Blunt Operating Scissor

Sharp/Sharp Operating Scissor

Proper Name: Sharp/Sharp Operating Scissor

Other Names: Sharp/Sharp, Nurse's Scissor, Suture Scissors, O.R. Scissors

Similar Instruments with Same Inspections: Iris

Length: 4.5", 5", 5.5", 6", and 6.5"

Surgical Use: Cutting and dissecting tissue and cutting surgical drapes

Tray Assembly Tips: Keep rings slightly separated and tips of scissors going in same direction

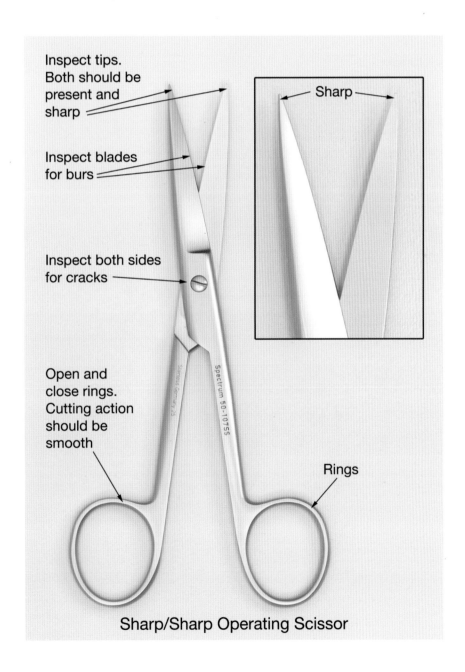

Inspect tips. Both should be present and sharp

Sharp

Inspect blades for burs

Inspect both sides for cracks

Open and close rings. Cutting action should be smooth

Rings

Sharp/Sharp Operating Scissor

Blunt/Blunt Operating Scissor

Proper Name: Blunt/Blunt Operating Scissor

Other Names: Blunt/Blunt, Nurse's Scissor, Suture Scissor, O.R. Scissor

Similar Instruments with Same Inspections: Metzenbaum, Mayo

Length: 4.5", 5", 5.5", 6", and 6.5"

Surgical Use: Cutting and dissecting tissue and cutting surgical drapes

Tray Assembly Tips: Keep rings slightly separated and tips of scissors going in the same direction

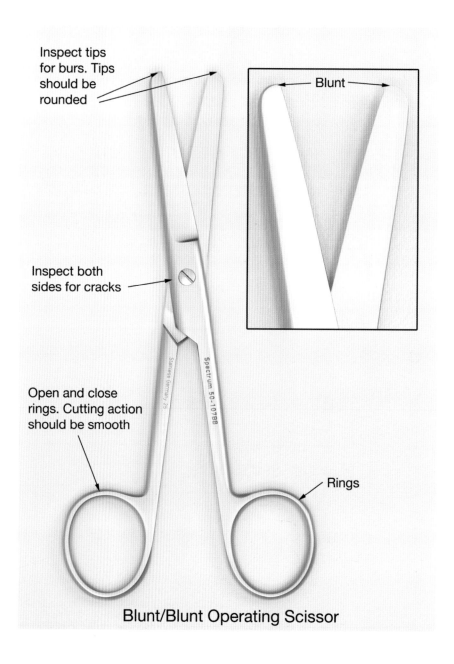

Inspect tips for burs. Tips should be rounded

Blunt

Inspect both sides for cracks

Open and close rings. Cutting action should be smooth

Rings

Blunt/Blunt Operating Scissor

Lister Bandage Scissor

Proper Name: Lister Bandage Scissor

Other Names: Bandage Scissor, Nurses Scissor

Similar Instruments with Same Inspections: Knowles, Hercules, Esmarch

Length: 5.5" and 7.5"

Criteria for Sharpness: Should be able to cut through a single layer of fabric or three layers of 4 X 4 gauze

Surgical Use: To cut bandages and dressings

Tray Assembly Tips: Keep rings slightly separated and tips of scissors going in same direction

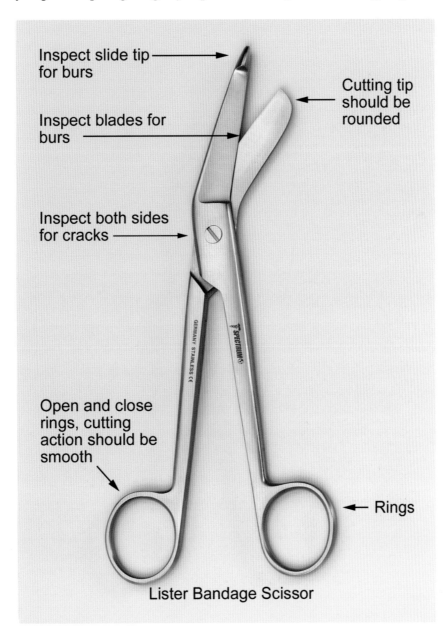

Inspect slide tip for burs

Cutting tip should be rounded

Inspect blades for burs

Inspect both sides for cracks

Open and close rings, cutting action should be smooth

Rings

Lister Bandage Scissor

Knowles Bandage Scissor

Proper Name: Knowles Bandage Scissor

Other Names: Straight Lister

Similar Instruments with Same Inspection: Lister Bandage Scissor

Blade Definition: Two straight blades with one blade having a bulbous tip

Length: 5.5"

Surgical Use: To cut bandages

Sharpness Test Standard: A single thickness of fabric

Tray Assembly Tips: Keep rings slightly separated and tips of scissors going in same direction

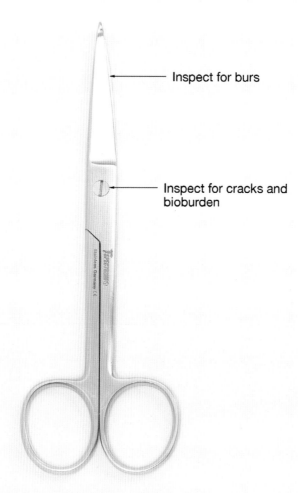

Inspect for burs

Inspect for cracks and bioburden

Knowles Bandage Scissor

Roger Wire Scissor

Proper Name: Roger Wire Scissor

Other Names: Wire Cutter, Angled Wire Cutter

Jaw Definition: Two angled blades with one blade having serrations

Length: 4.5"

Surgical Use: Cutting surgical wire

Sharpness Test Standard: The ability to cut fine surgical wire

Tray Assembly Tips: Keep rings slightly separated and tips of scissors going in same direction

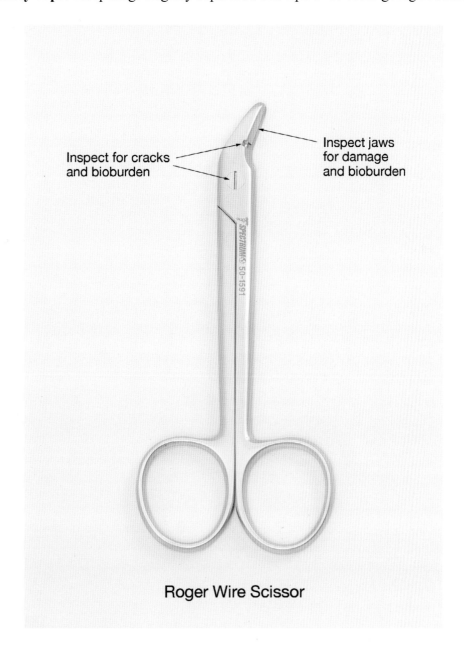

Roger Wire Scissor

Utility Scissor

Proper Name: Utility Scissor

Other Names: Paramedic Shear, Plastic Handled Scissor

Similar Instruments with Same Inspection: Any bandage scissor

Blade Definition: Serrated scissor blades with a plastic, bulbous tip

Length: 5.5", 7.5", 8.5"

Surgical Use: To cut bandages

Sharpness Test Standard: A single thickness of fabric

Tray Assembly Tips: Keep rings slightly separated and tips of scissors going in same direction

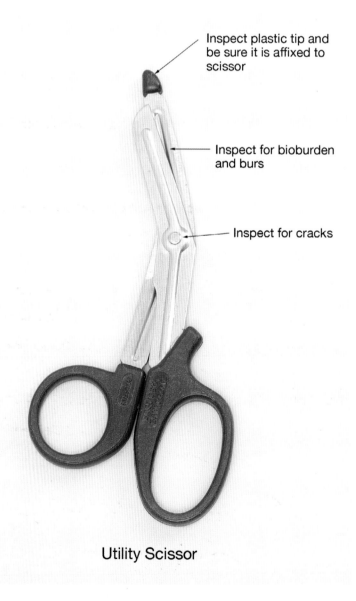

Utility Scissor

Iris Scissor

Proper Name: Iris Scissor

Other Names: Plastic Scissor, Small Sharp/Sharp, Eye Suture Scissor

Similar Instruments with Same Inspections: Goldman Fox, Bonn, Knapp, LaGrange

Length: 4.5" straight and curved most popular, 3.5" and 4"

  Most popular: 3.5" and 4"

Surgical Use: Very fine tissue dissection and cutting of fine suture

Sharpness Test Standard: Yellow scissor test material

Tray Assembly Tips: Due to fragile nature of distal tips, the use of tip protectors is advised

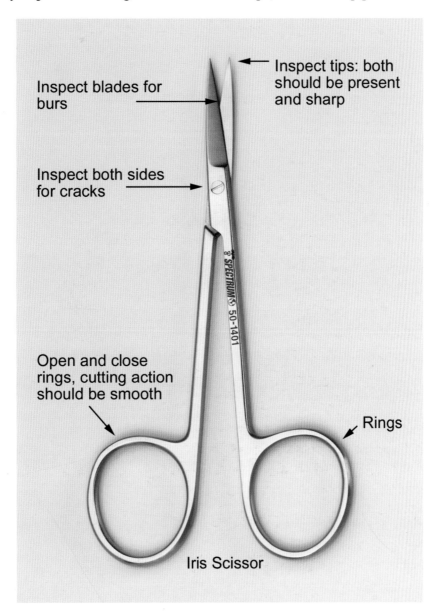

Inspect tips: both should be present and sharp

Inspect blades for burs

Inspect both sides for cracks

Open and close rings, cutting action should be smooth

Rings

Iris Scissor

Stevens Tenotomy Scissor

Proper Name: Stevens Tenotomy Scissor

Other Names: Tenotomy Scissor, Stevens Scissor

Similar Instruments with Same Inspection: Westcott Scissor

Blade Definition: Blades taper from mid-blade to the point - sharp or blunt points

Length: 4" to 4.5"

Surgical Use: Ophthalmic, ENT, and plastic surgery tissue cutting

Sharpness Test Standard: Yellow scissor test material

Tray Assembly Tips: Keep rings slightly separated and tips of scissors going in same direction

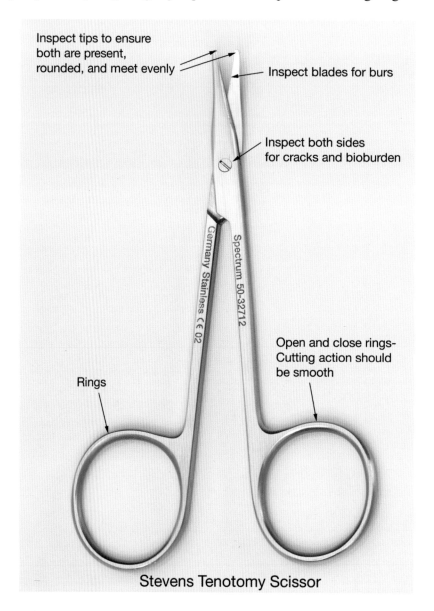

Inspect tips to ensure both are present, rounded, and meet evenly

Inspect blades for burs

Inspect both sides for cracks and bioburden

Germany Stainless CE 02

Spectrum 50-32712

Open and close rings-
Cutting action should be smooth

Rings

Stevens Tenotomy Scissor

Strabismus Scissor

Proper Name: Strabismus Scissor

Other Names: Blunt Scissor

Similar Instruments with Same Inspection: Iris Scissor, Metzenbaum Scissor

Blade Definition: Small, rounded, blunt blades

Length: 4"

Surgical Use: Ophthalmic, ENT, and plastic surgery dissection scissor

Sharpness Test Standard: Yellow scissor test material

Tray Assembly Tips: Keep rings slightly separated and tips of scissors going in same direction

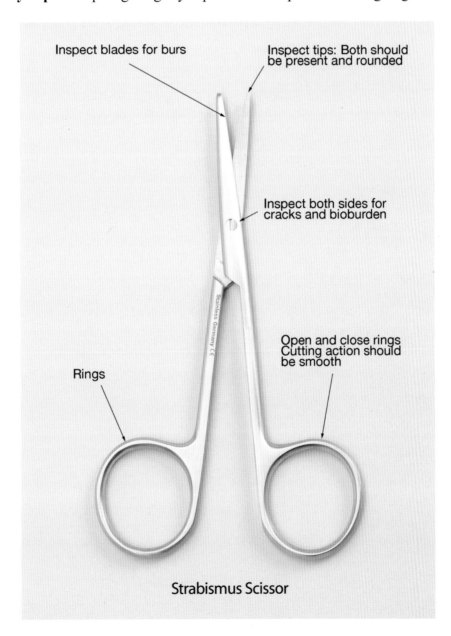

Inspect blades for burs

Inspect tips: Both should be present and rounded

Inspect both sides for cracks and bioburden

Rings

Open and close rings Cutting action should be smooth

Strabismus Scissor

Ribbon Iris

Proper Name: Ribbon Iris

Other Names: Big Ring Iris

Similar Instruments With Same Inspection: Any small dissection scissor

Blade Definition: Small pointed scissor blades

Length: 3.5", 4", 4.5"

Surgical Use: Fine dissection and cutting in plastic and ophthalmology surgery

Sharpness Test Standard: Yellow test material

Tray Assembly Tips: Keep rings slightly separated and tips of scissors going in same direction

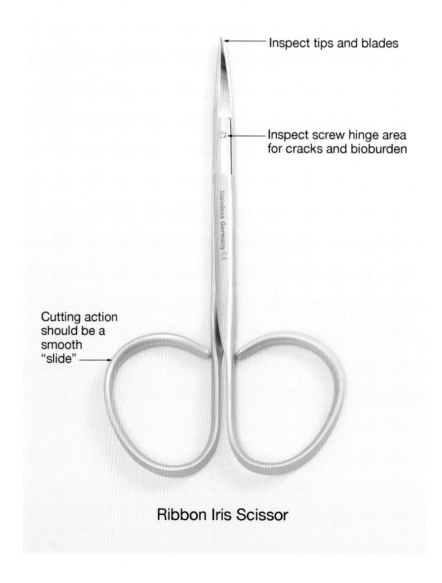

Inspect tips and blades

Inspect screw hinge area for cracks and bioburden

Cutting action should be a smooth "slide"

Ribbon Iris Scissor

Ribbon Tenotomy

Proper Name: Ribbon Tenotomy

Other Names: Big Ring Tenotomy

Similar Instruments With Same Inspection: Any other small dissection scissor

Blade Definition: Semi-pointed blades

Length: 3.5", 4", 4.5"

Surgical Use: Fine tissue dissection and cutting in plastic and ophthalmology surgery

Sharpness Test Standard: Yellow test material

Tray Assembly Tips: Keep rings slightly separated and tips of scissors going in same direction

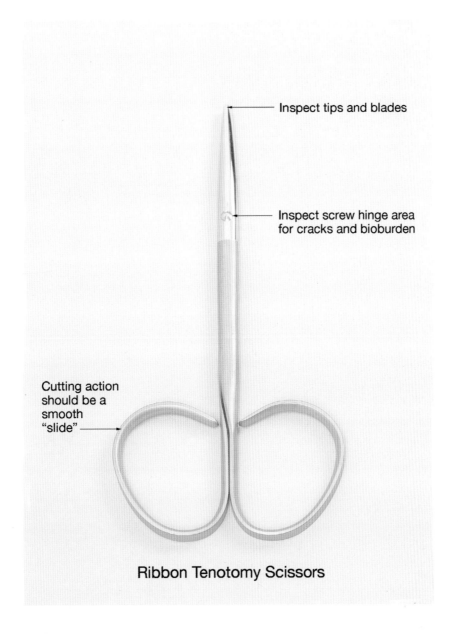

Inspect tips and blades

Inspect screw hinge area for cracks and bioburden

Cutting action should be a smooth "slide"

Ribbon Tenotomy Scissors

Littauer Stitch Scissor

Proper Name: Littauer Stitch Scissor

Other Names: Hook Scissor

Similar Instruments with Same Inspection: Spencer, Shortbent, Northbent

Blade Definition: Standard scissor blades with one blade that has a notch cut into it

Length: 3.5", 4.5", 5.5"

Surgical Use: The "notched" blade slides under suture to cut in the removal process

Sharpness Test Standard: Yellow test material on blades, suture strand on notch

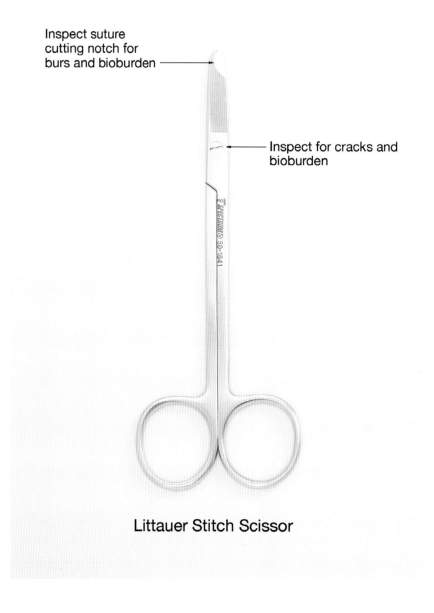

Inspect suture cutting notch for burs and bioburden

Inspect for cracks and bioburden

Littauer Stitch Scissor

Castroviejo Corneal Scissor

Proper Name: Castroviejo Corneal Scissor

Similar Instruments: Noyes, Barraquer, Westcott, McClure

Length: 4"

Surgical Use: To cut corneal tissue

Sharpness Test Standard: Yellow test material

Tray Assembly Tips: Keep rings slightly separated and tips of scissors going in same direction

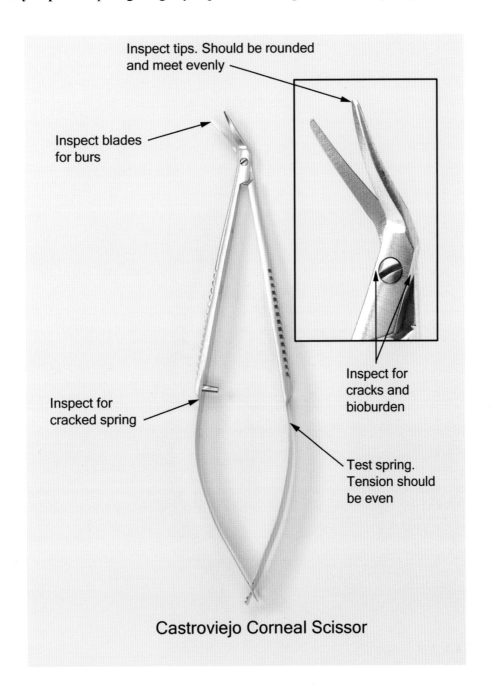

Inspect tips. Should be rounded and meet evenly

Inspect blades for burs

Inspect for cracks and bioburden

Inspect for cracked spring

Test spring. Tension should be even

Castroviejo Corneal Scissor

Littler Suture Scissor

Proper Name: Littler Suture Scissor

Other Names: Suture Carrying Scissor

Similar Instruments with Same Inspection: Ragnell Scissor

Blade Definition: Curved or straight blades with holes in each blade

Length: 4.5"

Surgical Use: For dissection and suture manipulation in plastic surgery

Sharpness Test Standard: Yellow scissor test material

Tray Assembly Tips: Keep rings slightly separated and tips of scissors going in same direction

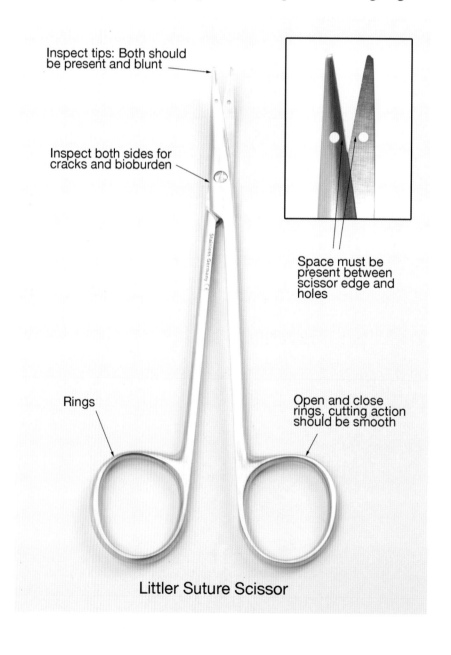

Inspect tips: Both should be present and blunt

Inspect both sides for cracks and bioburden

Space must be present between scissor edge and holes

Rings

Open and close rings, cutting action should be smooth

Littler Suture Scissor

Sims Uterine Scissor

Proper Name: Sims Uterine Scissor

Other Names: Uterine Scissor

Similar Instruments with Same Inspection: Kelly Uterine Scissor, Mayo Uterine Scissor

Blade Definition: Two scissor blades with sharp/sharp points, sharp/blunt points, or blunt/blunt points

Length: 8"

Surgical Use: To cut the uterus

Sharpness Test Standard: Red test material

Tray Assembly Tips: Keep rings slightly separated and tips of scissors going in same direction

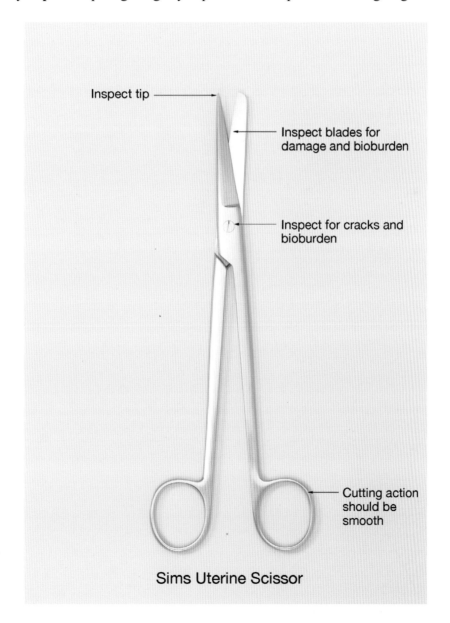

Inspect tip

Inspect blades for damage and bioburden

Inspect for cracks and bioburden

Cutting action should be smooth

Sims Uterine Scissor

Braun Episiotomy Scissor

Proper Name: Braun Episiotomy Scissor

Similar Instruments with Same Inspection: None

Length: 5.5" and 8.5"

Tip Definition: Very blunt scissor blade tips

Surgical Use: Used for vaginal delivery

Sharpness Test Standard: Red test material

Tray Assembly Tips: Sterilize with rings open

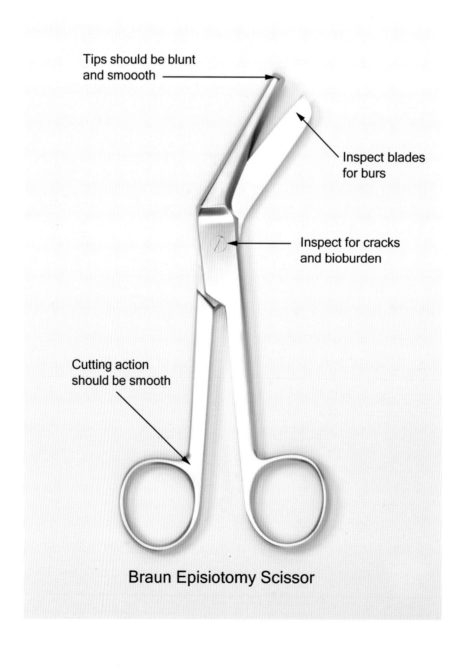

Tips should be blunt and smoooth

Inspect blades for burs

Inspect for cracks and bioburden

Cutting action should be smooth

Braun Episiotomy Scissor

Caplan Nasal Bone Scissor

Proper Name: Caplan Nasal Bone Scissor

Other Names: Angled Nasal Scissor

Similar Instruments with Same Inspection: McIndoe Bone Cutting Forcep, Kazanjian Nasal Cutting Forcep

Blade Definition: Serrated blades with double action and angled design

Length: 8"

Surgical Use: Cutting of nasal bone and cartilage

Sharpness Test Standard: Red scissor test material

Tray Assembly Tips: Keep rings slightly separated and tips of scissors going in same direction

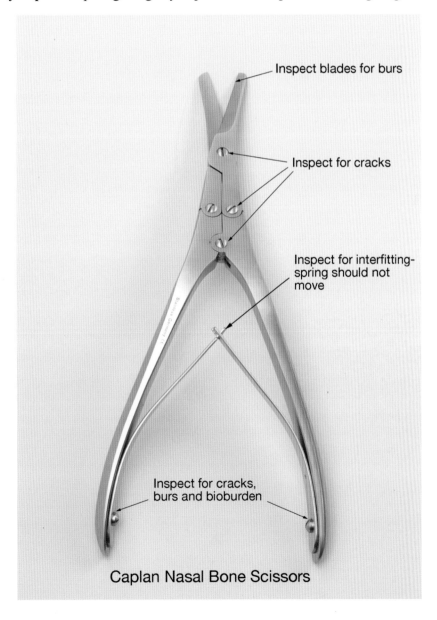

Inspect blades for burs

Inspect for cracks

Inspect for interfitting-spring should not move

Inspect for cracks, burs and bioburden

Caplan Nasal Bone Scissors

Cottle Dorsal Scissor

Proper Name: Cottle Dorsal Scissor

Other Names: Angled Scissor, Angled Mayo

Similar Instruments with Same Inspection: Fomon Scissor

Blade Definition: Round blades

Length: 5.5" and 6.5"

Surgical Use: Nasal dissection procedures

Sharpness Test Standard: Red scissor test material

Tray Assembly Tips: Keep rings slightly separated and tips of scissors going in same direction

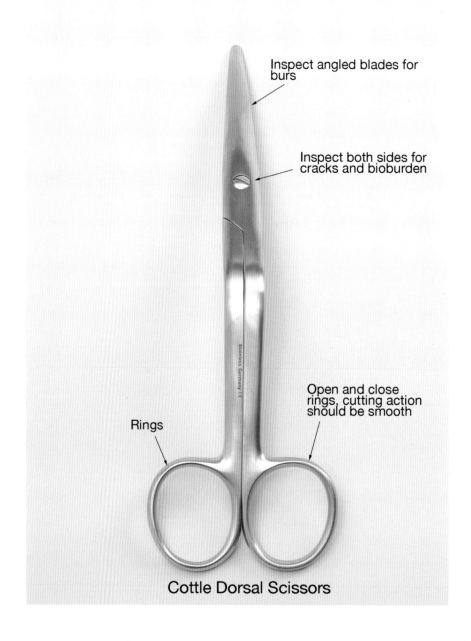

Inspect angled blades for burs

Inspect both sides for cracks and bioburden

Open and close rings, cutting action should be smooth

Rings

Cottle Dorsal Scissors

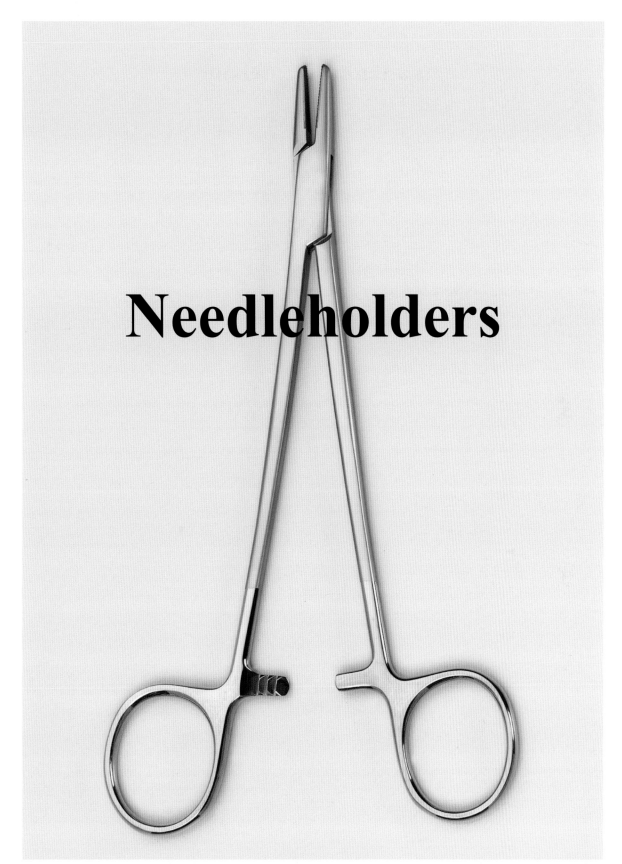

Needleholders

Needleholders – designed to drive suture needles to close or rejoin a wound or surgical site.

Facts about Needleholders

- All needleholder jaws wear out
- All needleholder jaws wear out at the tips of the jaws first
- All needleholders crack in the box lock area or the jaw area
- Only gold handled needleholder jaws can be replaced
- Needleholders should never be sterilized with ratchets clicked and/or engaged

Gold Rings: Indicate the jaw portion contains tungsten carbide inserts. The needleholder is made out of stainless steel. The gripping portion of the jaws have two pieces (inserts) made out of the metal tungsten carbide. The tungsten carbide inserts are a harder metal than stainless steel. The advantages of tungsten carbide jaws are:

1. They will not wear out as fast as stainless steel.
2. They grip the suture needle more precisely with less slippage.
3. When the jaws wear out the inserts can simply be replaced.

Non-Gold Rings: Indicate the jaws are made out of the same material (stainless steel) as the rest of the needleholder. This design of needleholder will wear out faster and the jaws cannot be replaced.

Points of Inspection

- **Jaws:** Inspect serrations for wear, cracked or missing inserts, and worn or chipped edges. Inspect jaws for dark colored bioburden and stains. If the needleholder has smooth jaws, close the ratchets all the way and the hold needleholder up to light. If you can see light between the jaw tips, this needleholder is in need of repair.
- **Neck:** Inspect for cracks.
- **Box Lock:** Inspect for cracks on both sides. Also inspect for blood and baked on bioburden.
- **Shanks:** Should be straight.
- **Ratchet:** Test ratchet by opening and closing. This action should be precise and smooth. With needleholder ratchets closed completely, all edges should meet evenly.

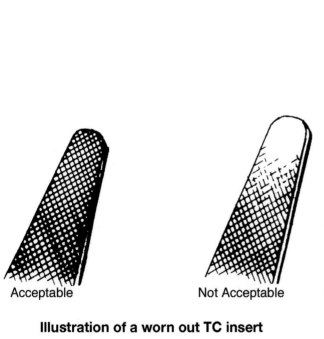

Acceptable   Not Acceptable

Illustration of a worn out TC insert

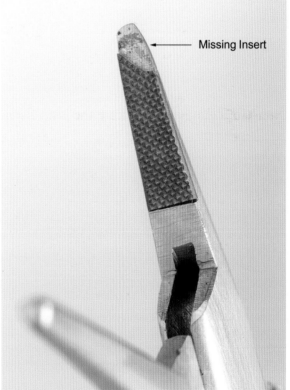

Missing Insert

Advantages of Gold Handled Needleholders

- Grips the suture needle more firmly

- Does not wear out as quickly

- Can be easily re-jawed/restored by your repair vendor

Post Operative Care: Open the instrument by separating the rings or ratchet. Never allow blood to dry onto instruments. To prevent blood from drying onto instruments, soak in an enzymatic solution or place a moist towel saturated with water over the instruments.

Cleaning Instructions: Follow standard decontamination procedures, followed by terminal sterilization procedures.

Tray Assembly Tips: Sterilize instrument with ratchets open.

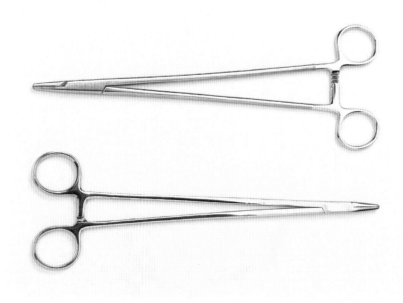

Gold handled Needleholder with replaceable Tungsten Carbide jaws
Bottom – Standard Needleholder; jaws cannot be replaced

Needleholder Jaw Inspection

All needleholder jaws will wear out the tread in normal suturing. Gold handle needleholder jaws are made of tungsten carbide and can be replaced. Standard needleholder jaws (those without gold handles) cannot be replaced.

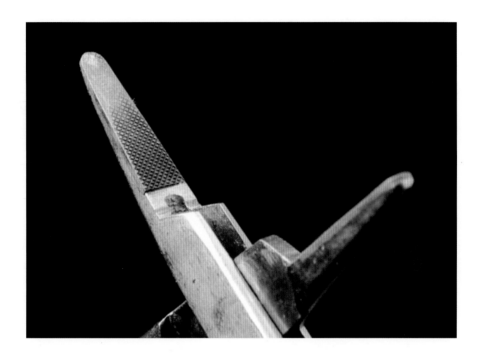

Worn out Tungsten Carbide jaw

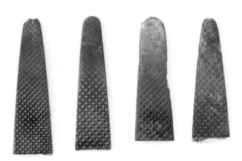

Worn out jaws

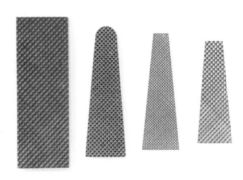

New jaws

Jaw Inspection

If any bioburden or discoloration is discovered on the jaw or box lock, the instrument must be reprocessed through decontamination. A stiff brush will most likely remove the bioburden. If it's not clean, it can't be sterile. It is not appropriate to clean instruments at the assembly table.

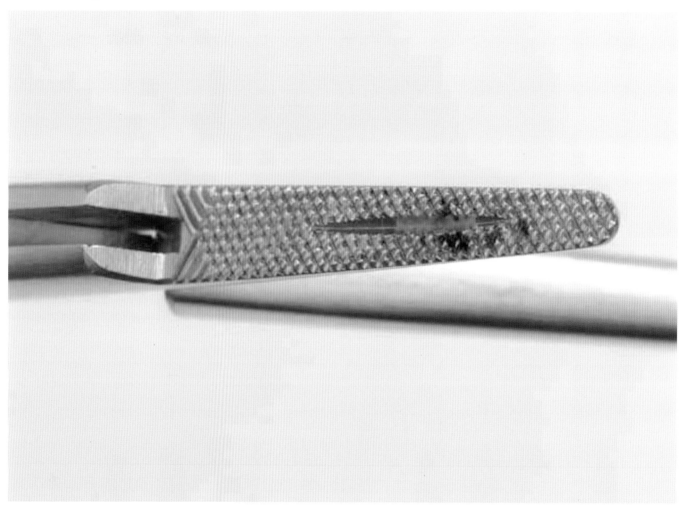

Inspecting Diamond Dusted Microvascular Needleholders

Jaw wear is an issue with all types of needleholders. Diamond Dusting is a process that enables the Needleholder to grip very fine suture needles. This agitated metal surface does, however, wear smooth as illustrated in the photos below. Microvascular needleholders should be inspected prior to tray assembly.

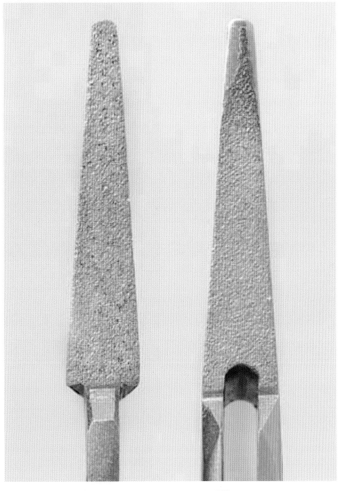

Good　　　　**Worn**

Diamond Dusted Needleholders

Sternum Wire Twister

Due to the pressure of stainless steel wire being twisted, the jaws of wire twisters are susceptible to cracking. This malfunction allows pieces of the tungsten carbide jaw to drop into the surgical site. Inspect the jaws prior to tray assembly and if pieces are missing or jaw wear is visible, do not use the instrument. Schedule the wire twister for repair.

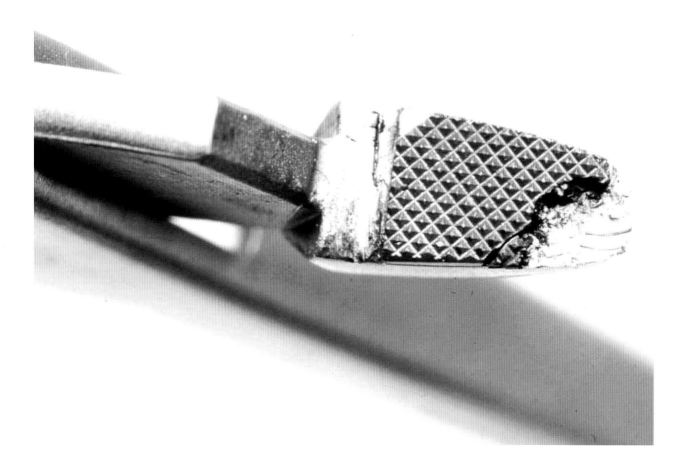

Webster Needleholder

Proper Name: Webster Needleholder

Jaw Description: Serrated most common smooth available

Length: 5"

Surgical Use: For driving suture needles

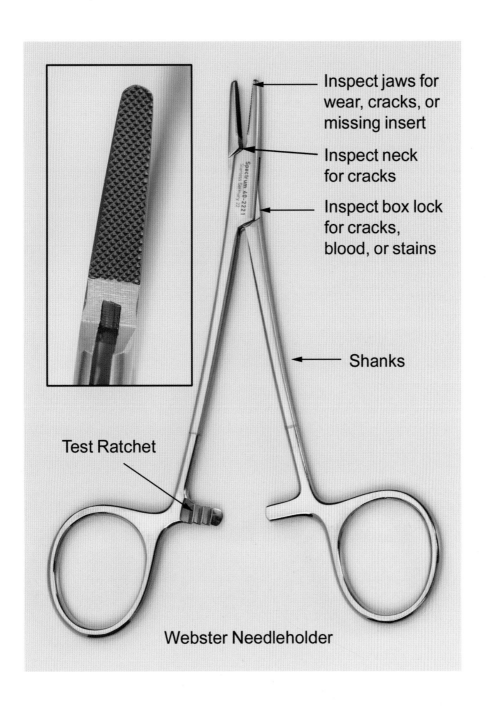

Inspect jaws for wear, cracks, or missing insert

Inspect neck for cracks

Inspect box lock for cracks, blood, or stains

Shanks

Test Ratchet

Webster Needleholder

Halsey Needleholder

Proper Name: Halsey Needleholder

Jaw Description: Smooth or serrated jaws equally popular

Length: 5"

Surgical Use: For driving suture needles

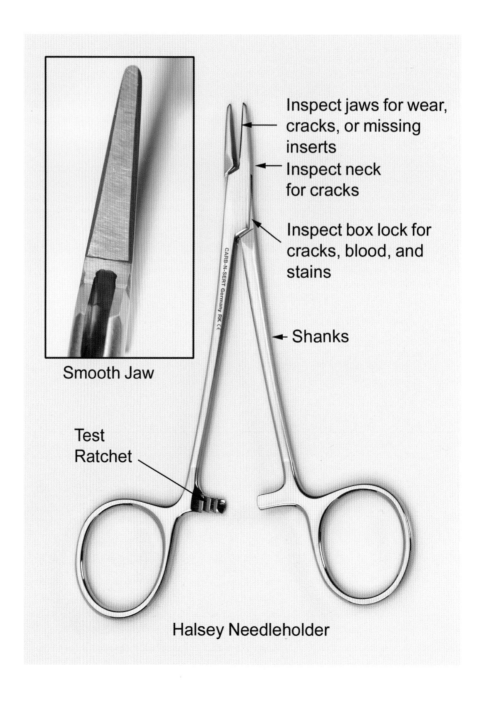

Smooth Jaw

Inspect jaws for wear, cracks, or missing inserts

Inspect neck for cracks

Inspect box lock for cracks, blood, and stains

Shanks

Test Ratchet

Halsey Needleholder

Derf Needleholder

Proper Name: Derf Needleholder

Jaw Description: Serrated jaws

Length: 5"

Surgical Use: For driving suture needles

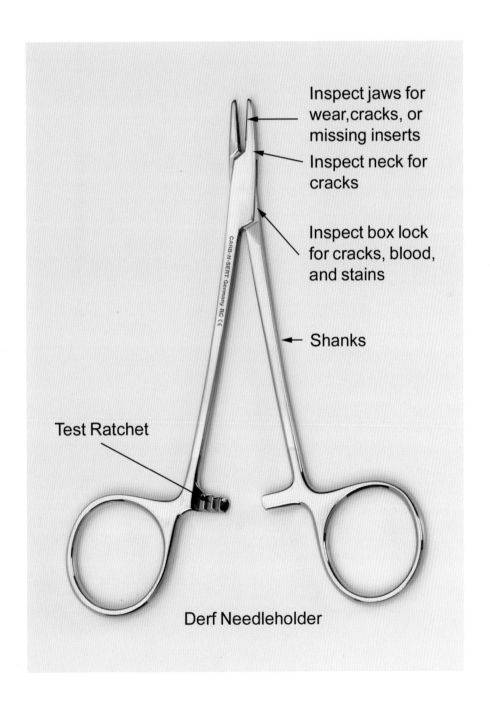

Inspect jaws for wear,cracks, or missing inserts

Inspect neck for cracks

Inspect box lock for cracks, blood, and stains

Shanks

Test Ratchet

Derf Needleholder

Mayo Hegar Needleholder

Proper Name: Mayo Hegar Needleholder

Jaw Description: Serrated jaws

Length: 6", 7", 8", 9", 10", 12"

Surgical Use: For driving suture needles

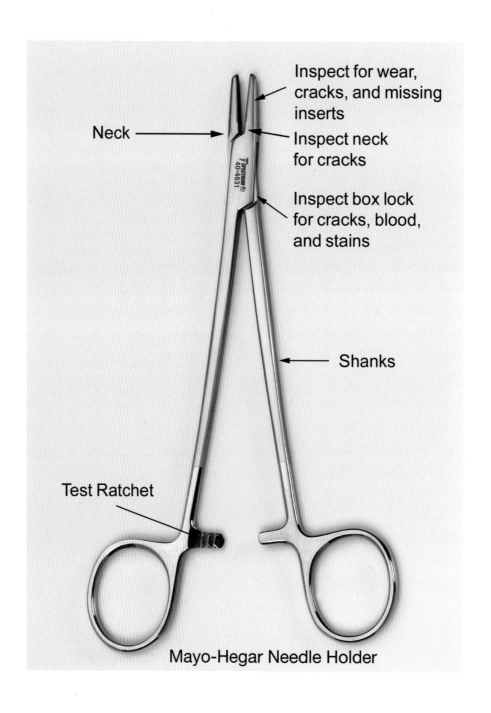

Neck

Inspect for wear, cracks, and missing inserts

Inspect neck for cracks

Inspect box lock for cracks, blood, and stains

Shanks

Test Ratchet

Mayo-Hegar Needle Holder

Crilewood Needleholder

Proper Name: Crilewood Needleholder

Jaw Description: Serrated jaws

Length: 6", 7", 8", 9", 10", 11", 12"

Surgical Use: For driving suture needles

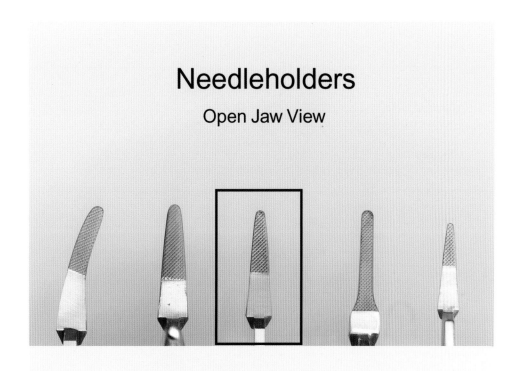

Needleholders
Open Jaw View

Needleholders
Closed Jaw View

Heaney   Mayo Hegar   Crilewood   Ryder   Micro-Vascular

Heaney Needleholder

Proper Name: Heaney Needleholder

Jaw Description: Curved, serrated jaws

Length: 8"

Jaw Definitions: Curved

Surgical Use: For driving suture needles

Needleholders
Open Jaw View

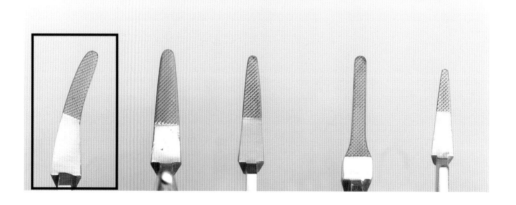

Needleholders
Closed Jaw View

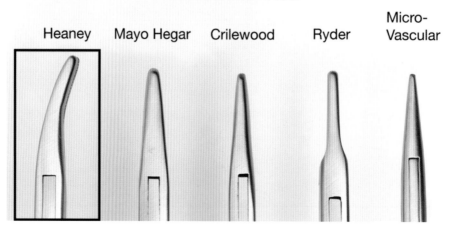

| Heaney | Mayo Hegar | Crilewood | Ryder | Micro-Vascular |

Ryder Needleholder

Proper Name: Ryder Needleholder

Jaw Description: Serrated

Length: 6", 7", 8", 9", 10"

Surgical Use: For driving suture needles

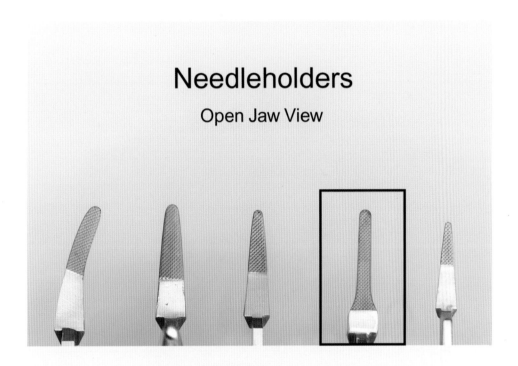

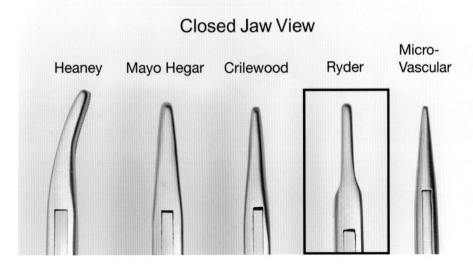

Olsen Hegar Needleholder

Proper Name: Olsen Hegar Needleholder

Jaw Description: Serrated jaws with a scissor built in above box lock area

Length: 4.5", 5.5", 6.5", 7.5"

Surgical Use: For driving suture needles

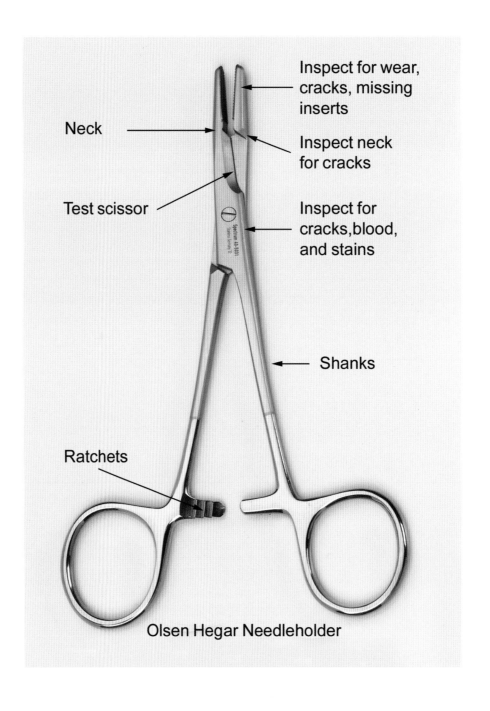

Inspect for wear, cracks, missing inserts

Neck

Inspect neck for cracks

Test scissor

Inspect for cracks, blood, and stains

Shanks

Ratchets

Olsen Hegar Needleholder

Castroviejo Needleholder

Proper Name: Castroviejo Needleholder

Jaw Description: Smooth or serrated. Due to its delicate nature, it is recommended that this instrument be stored in a protective case.

Length: 5.5", 7", 8.5"

Surgical Use: For driving small suture needles

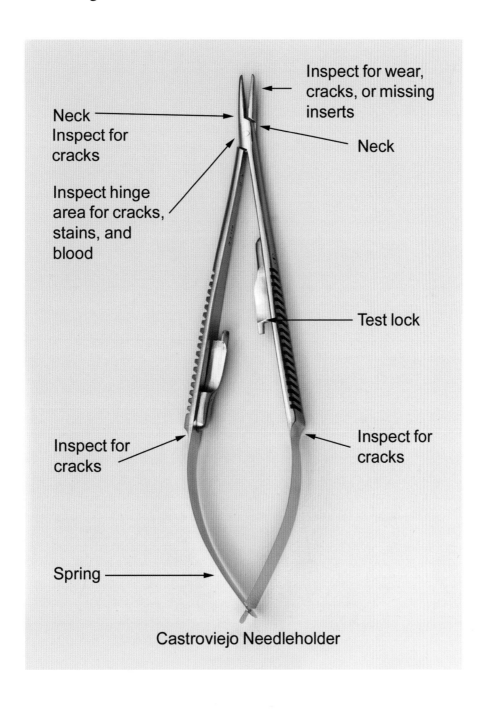

Castroviejo Needleholder

Suction Devices

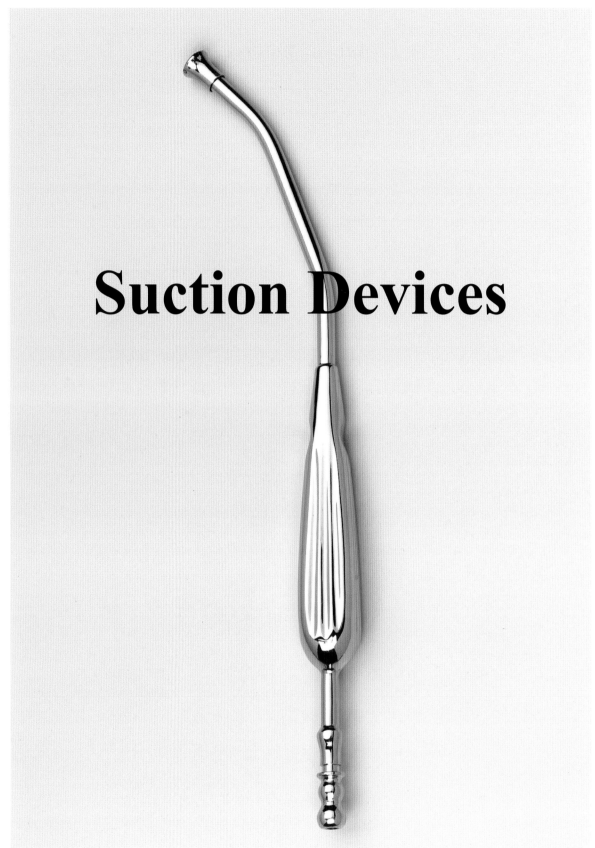

Suction Devices – used to extract blood and solutions out of a surgical site.

Suction Devices

Points of Inspection:

- **Tips:** Inspect for sharp edges, dents and trapped surgical debris.
- **Shaft:** Inspect for dents due to bending.
- **Suction Control:** Inspect that tubing union has proper soldering and that there is no breakdown of the union.
- **Stylet:** Should be able to insert at proximal end. Should not be inserted during sterilization process.

Cleaning Instructions: Use a cleaning brush that enters and completely exits suction device.

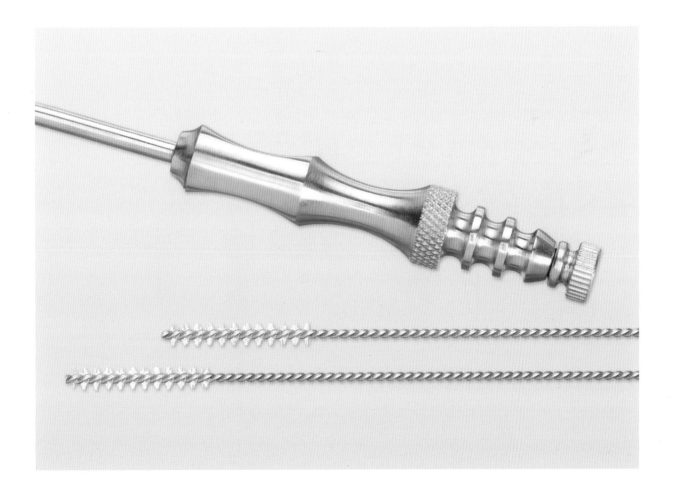

Baron Suction Tube

Proper Name: Baron Suction Tube

Size, Diameter: 3 French, 5 French, 7 French

Length: 7.5cm

Tray Assembly Tips: Always include stylet

Surgical Use: Removal of ENT fluids

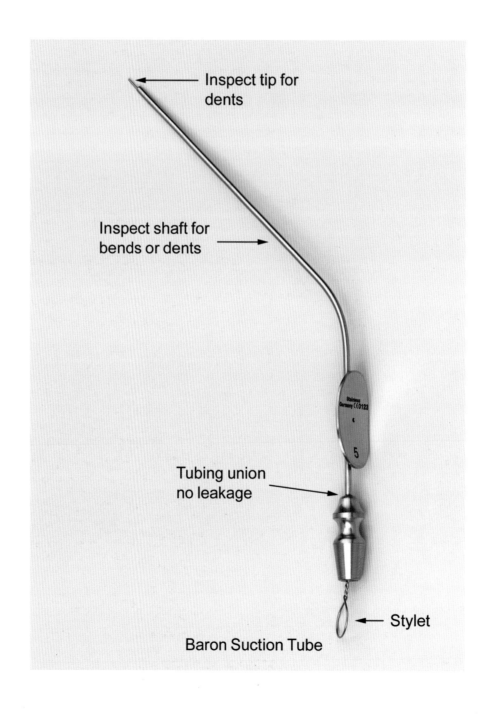

Inspect tip for dents

Inspect shaft for bends or dents

Tubing union no leakage

Stylet

Baron Suction Tube

Frazier Suction Tube

Proper Name: Frazier Suction Tube

Other Names: Neuro Suction, Nasal Suction

Size, Diameter: 6, 8, 10, 12, 14 French

Length: 7"

Tray Assembly Tips: Always include stylet

Surgical Use: Removal of ENT and neuro fluids

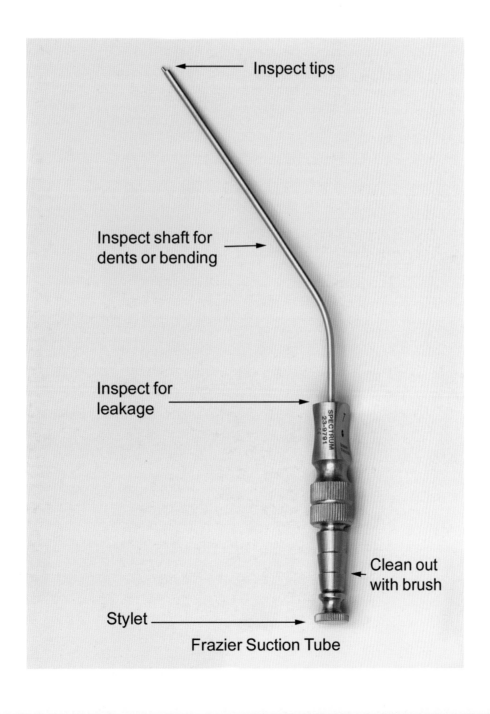

Inspect tips

Inspect shaft for dents or bending

Inspect for leakage

Clean out with brush

Stylet

Frazier Suction Tube

Yankauer Suction Tube

Proper Name: Yankauer Suction Tube

Other Names: Tonsil Tip, Sucker, Tonsillar Suction

Size, Diameter: Standard

Length: 12"

Post Operative Care: Disassemble and rinse with enzymatic solution or water

Tray Assembly Tips: Be sure tip and connector are secure

Surgical Use: Removal of fluids

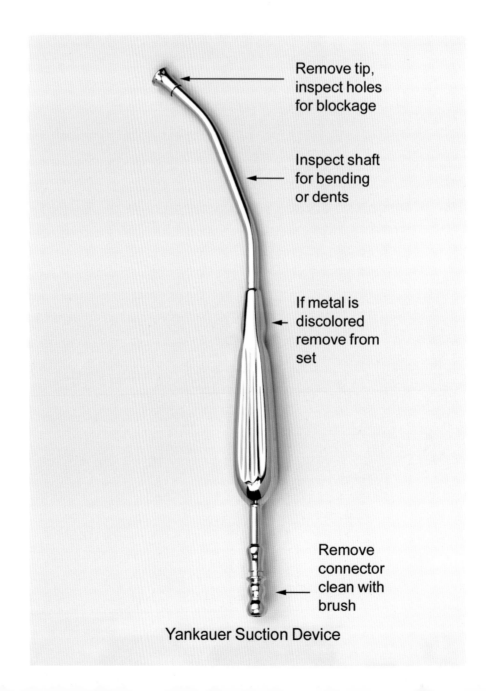

Remove tip, inspect holes for blockage

Inspect shaft for bending or dents

If metal is discolored remove from set

Remove connector clean with brush

Yankauer Suction Device

Poole Suction Tube

Proper Name: Poole Suction Tube

Size, Diameter: 23 French Angled, 30 French Angled

Length: 9"

Post Operative Care: Disassemble and rinse with enzymatic solution or water

Tray Assembly Tips: Sterilize disassembled

Surgical Use: Removal of fluids from surgical site

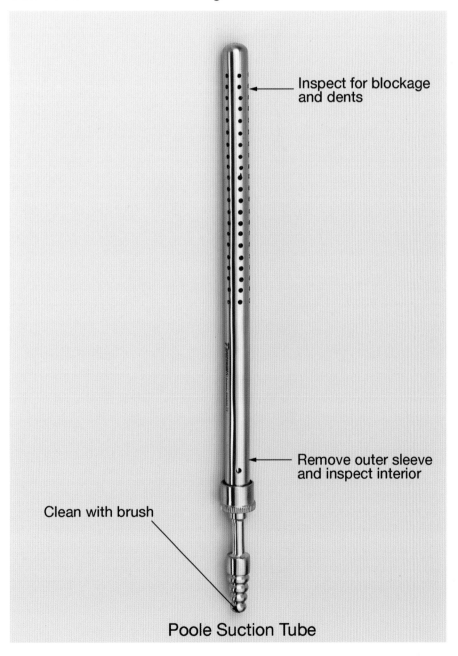

Inspect for blockage and dents

Remove outer sleeve and inspect interior

Clean with brush

Poole Suction Tube

Intercardiac Suction Device

Proper Name: Intercardiac Suction Device

Other Names: Cardiac Suction, Pemco

Size, Diameter: Standard

Length: 10.5", Junior size 7"

Post Operative Care: Disassemble and rinse with enzymatic solution or water

Tray Assembly Tips: Be sure all tips are present

Surgical Use: Cardiac procedures, and removal of fluids

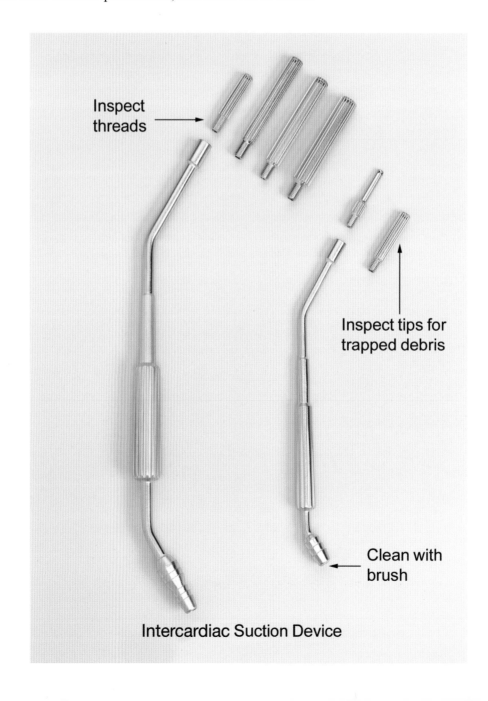

Intercardiac Suction Device

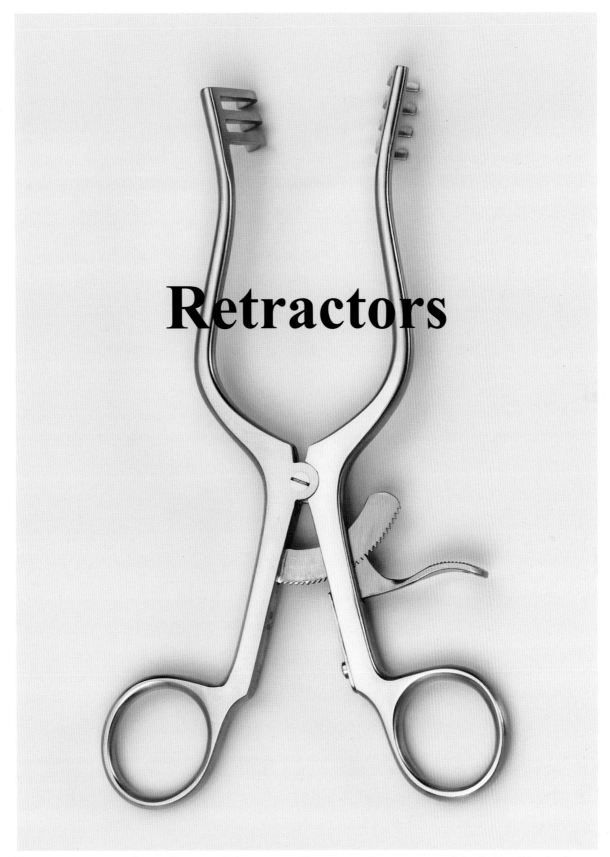

Retractors

Retractors – primarily used to move tissue and organs aside in order to keep them exposed throughout surgery.

Paper Test for Retractors

Very old surgical instruments' metal finish can and will flake off. The first indication of this wear is the appearance of the metal surface (see photo below). To determine if a finish is unstable, (which may result in metal particles dropping off into the surgical site), follow the steps below:

1) Put on a pair of examination gloves
2) Hold the instrument above a white piece of paper
3) Aggressively rub the instrument with your gloved hands
4) Examine the piece of paper for metal flakes
5) If there are flakes on the paper, remove the instrument immediately and discontinue use

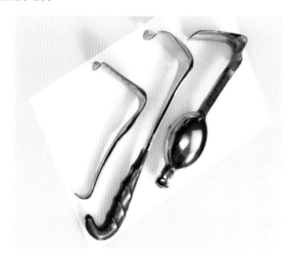

Points of Inspection

- **Distal ends:** Inspect for bent blades/prongs
- **Release lever**: Flick release lever, it should spring back into place and open and close smoothly
- **Screw:** Inspect for cracks
- **Spring area:** Inspect for cracks

Abdominal Flexible Retractor System

Proper Name: Abdominal Flexible Retractor System

Other Names: Bookwalter™

     This table-mounted retractor system offers great choices to the surgeon for deep abdominal retraction. The set contains various retractor blades consisting of fixed blades and malleable blades. The blades attach to either a standard ratchet or tilt ratchet. The ratchets then attach to the retractor ring, which comes in various sizes and shapes. The oval rings attach to bars, which attach to the main table post.

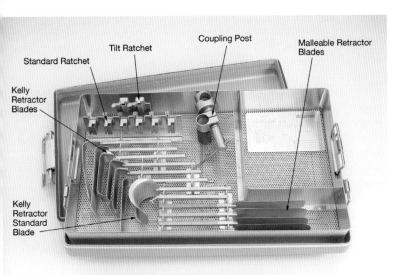

Flexible Abdominal Retractor System Tray 1

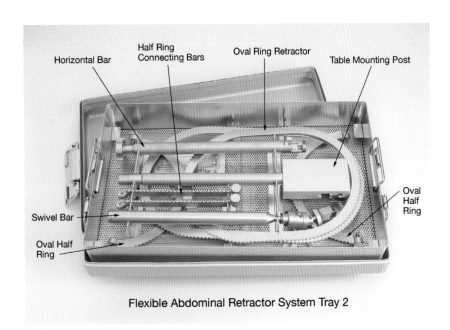

Flexible Abdominal Retractor System Tray 2

Flexible Abdominal Retractor Blade

Proper Name: Flexible Abdominal Retractor Blade

Other Names: Kelly, Richardson, Bookwalter Blade, Malleable Blades

Similar Instruments with Same Inspection: Retractor Blades

Blade Definition: Flat, bendable stainless steel

Length: 8", 10", 12"

Width: 2", 3", 4", 5"

Surgical Use: Attaches to a table-mounted abdominal retractor system and performs deep cavity retraction.

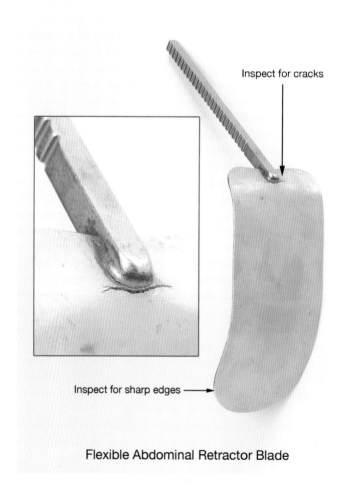

Inspect for cracks

Inspect for sharp edges

Flexible Abdominal Retractor Blade

Flexible Abdominal Retractor Ratchets

Proper Name: Flexible Abdominal Retractor Ratchets

Other Names: Tilt Ratchet, Standard Ratchet

Similar Instruments with Same Inspection: Bookwalter™ Ratchets

Surgical Use: Holds retractor blades in place while attached to retractor ring

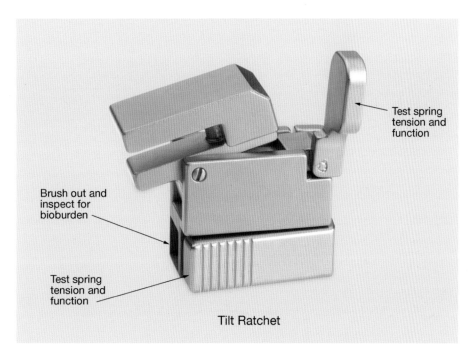

Test spring tension and function

Brush out and inspect for bioburden

Test spring tension and function

Tilt Ratchet

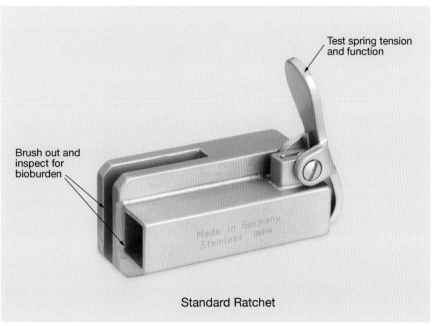

Test spring tension and function

Brush out and inspect for bioburden

Standard Ratchet

Weitlaner Retractor

Proper Name: Weitlaner Retractor

Other Names: Self-retaining rake, Spreader

Type: Self-Retaining

Size: 4.5", 5.5", 6.5", 7.5", 8", sharp or blunt prongs

Surgical Use: Retaining of shallow tissue in orthopedic and neurological cases

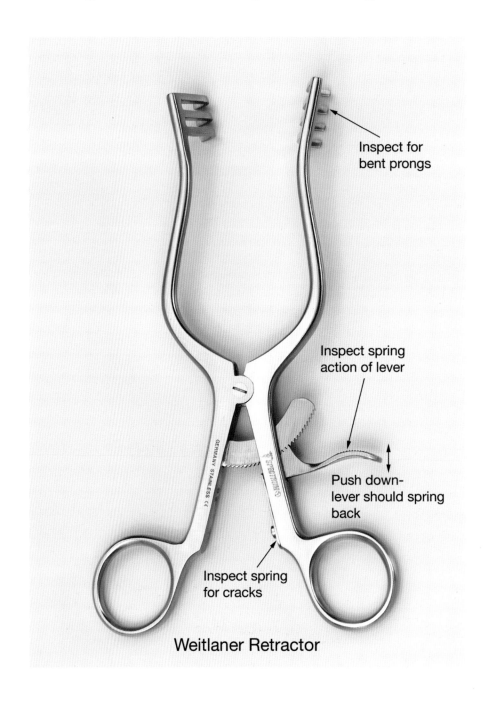

Inspect for bent prongs

Inspect spring action of lever

Push down-lever should spring back

Inspect spring for cracks

Weitlaner Retractor

100

Gelpi Retractor

Proper Name: Gelpi Retractor

Type: Self-Retaining

Size: 3.5", 4.5", 5.5", and 7" with sharp singular prongs

SHARPS RISK. The use of a tip protector on distal sharp prongs is recommended

Surgical Use: Retracts tissue at various depths

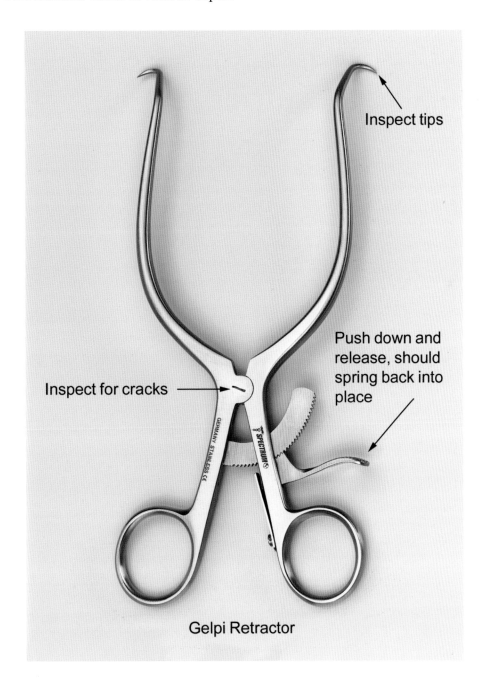

Inspect tips

Push down and release, should spring back into place

Inspect for cracks

Gelpi Retractor

Senn Retractor

Proper Name: Senn Retractor

Other Names: Rakes, Mueller

Type: Hand-held

Size: 6.5", sharp or blunt prongs

Tray Assembly Tips: The use of a tip protector on distal sharp prongs is recommended

Surgical Use: Retracts skin in small incisions

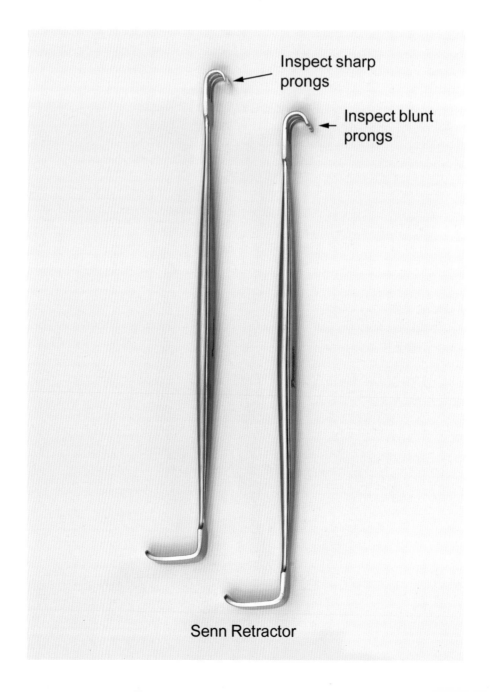

Inspect sharp prongs

Inspect blunt prongs

Senn Retractor

Army-Navy Retractor

Proper Name: Army-Navy Retractor

Other Names: USA Retractor, US Army Retractor

Size: 8"

Tray Assembly Tips: Retractor is designed and used as a pair

Surgical Use: Tissue retraction

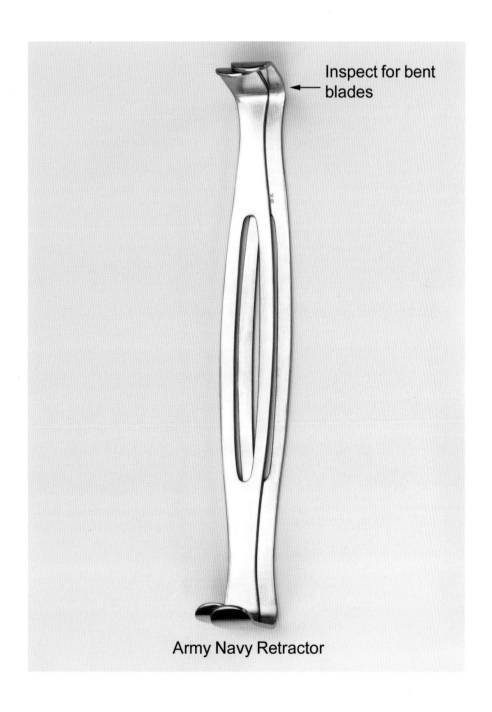

Inspect for bent blades

Army Navy Retractor

Richardson Retractor

Proper Name: Richardson Retractor

Handles: Two types: Loop and Hollow

Size: 9.5" with various width and depth of blade

Surgical Use: Deeper retraction of tissue

Kelly Retractor

Proper Name: Kelly Retractor

Other Name: Kelly Richardson, Large Richardson

Size: 10" Length, blade size is 2" larger

Compared with a Richardson retractor, the Kelly retractor is always the larger bladed retractor

Tray Assembly Tips: Kelly retractors are usually the largest and should be placed on the bottom of the tray

Surgical Use: Deep and wide retraction

Note: The only difference between a Richardson Retractor and a Kelly Retractor is the size of the blades - Kelly Retractors have larger blade dimensions

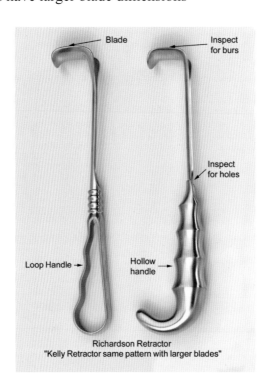

Richardson Retractor
"Kelly Retractor same pattern with larger blades"

Malleable Retractor

Proper Name: Malleable Retractor

Other Name: Ribbon

Size: 13" Length, .5", 1", 1.5", 2", 2.5", 3", 3.5" width

Tray Assembly Tips: Flatten out retractor and place retractor on side of tray

Surgical Use: Tissue retraction with a malleable blade can be formed into any shape to do the retraction

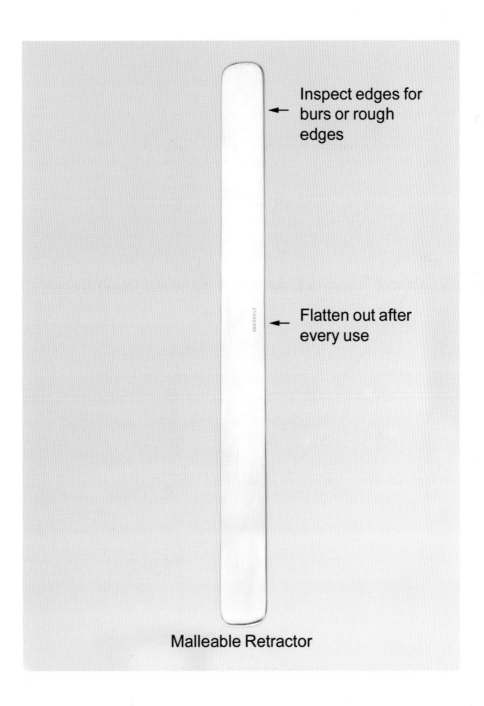

Inspect edges for burs or rough edges

Flatten out after every use

Malleable Retractor

Richardson-Eastman Retractor

Proper Name: Richardson-Eastman Retractor

Other Names: Richardsons

Similar Instruments with Same Inspection: Kelly Retractor

Blade Definition: Double ended blades

Length: 10" and 11"

Surgical Use: Retraction of tissue in surgical sites

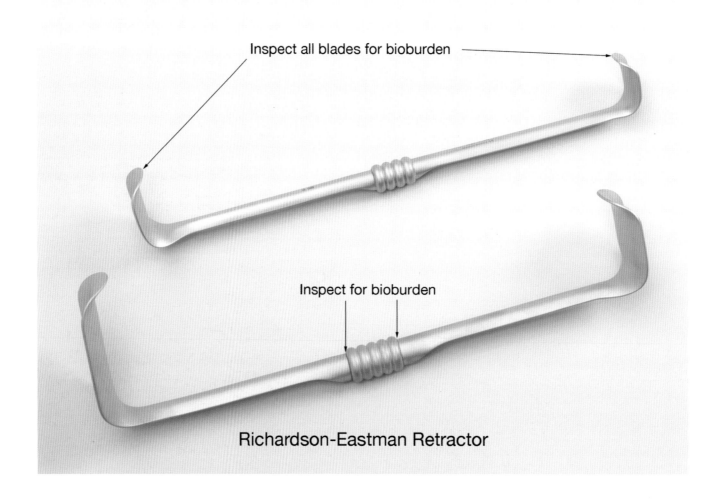

Inspect all blades for bioburden

Inspect for bioburden

Richardson-Eastman Retractor

Deaver Retractor

Proper Name: Deaver Retractor

Type: Hand Held

Size: Width: .375", .75", .5", 1", 1.5", 2", 3"- Length: 7", 8", 9", 12", 13"

Tray Assembly Tips: Deaver retractors belong on the bottom or side of tray

Surgical Use: Very deep tissue retraction

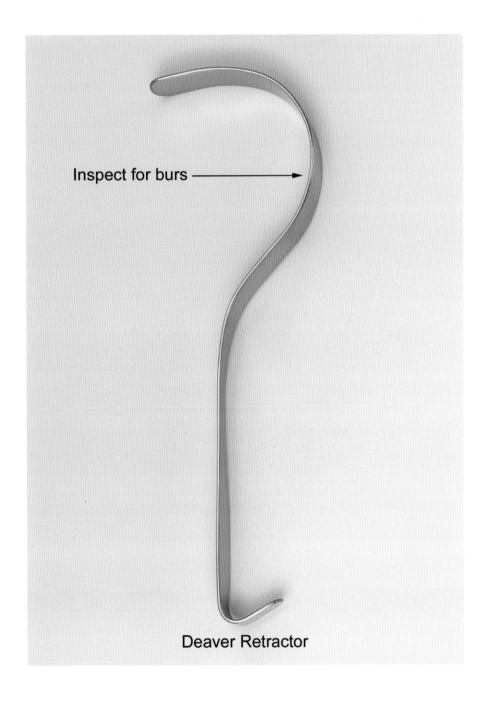

Inspect for burs ⟶

Deaver Retractor

Alm Retractor

Proper Name: Alm Retractor

Other Names: Little Spreader

Type: Self-Retaining

Size: 2.5" or 3.5"

Tray Assembly Tips: Small retractors should be placed on top of heavy instruments

Surgical Use: Small incisions

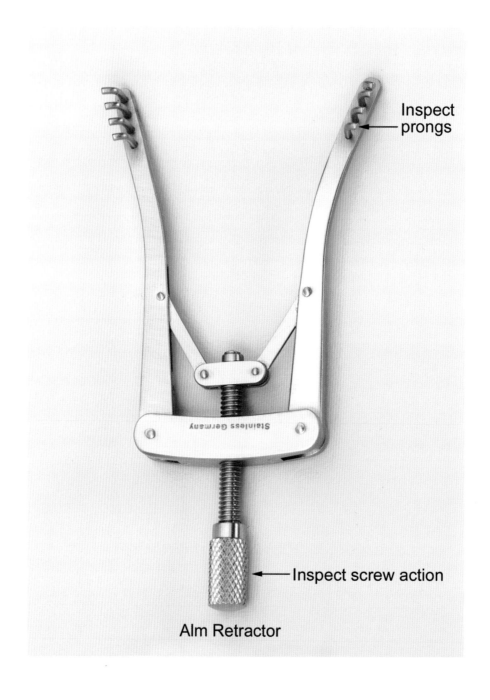

Alm Retractor

Balfour Retractor

Proper Name: Balfour Retractor

Type: Self retaining

Size: 7" spread with various sizes of center blades and side blades

Tray Assembly Tips: Make sure all blades, nuts, and attachments are in the tray

Surgical Use: Abdominal retraction

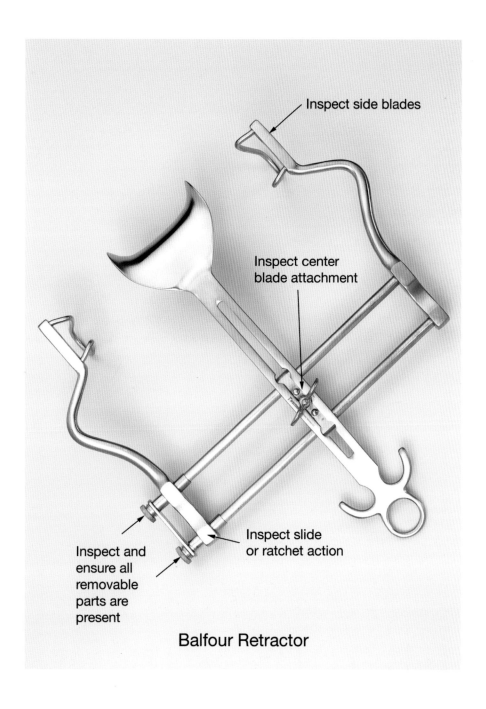

Balfour Retractor

Meyerding Finger Retractor

Proper Name: Meyerding Finger Retractor

Other Names: Ring Retractor, Finger Retractor

Similar Instruments with Same Inspection: Mathieu and Senn Retractor

Blade Definition: Solid angled blade or various teeth configurations and sizes available

Length: 7"

Surgical Use: Retraction of skin at small shallow surgical sites

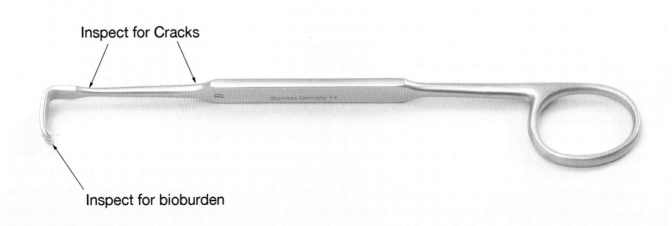

Inspect for Cracks

Inspect for bioburden

Meyerding Finger Retractor

Volkman Retractor

Proper Name: Volkman Retractor

Other Name: Rakes

Type: Hand-held

Size: 7.5" long with 2, 3, 4, 5, or 6 prongs - sharp or dull

Tray Assembly Tips: The use of a tip protector on distal sharp prongs is appropriate

Surgical Use: Small retraction for small incisions

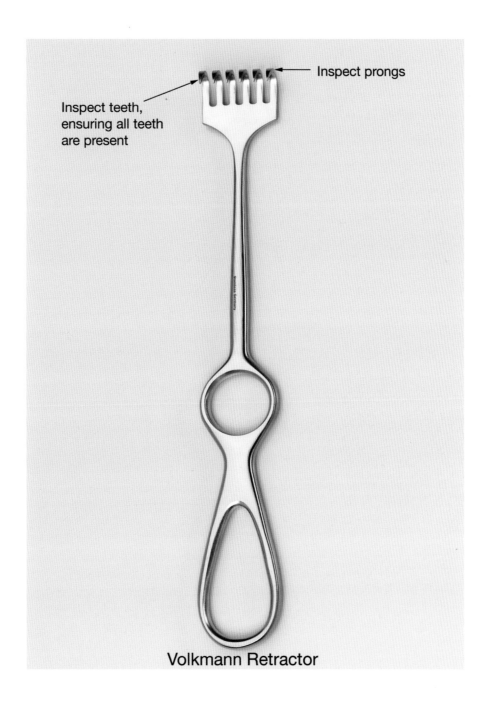

Inspect prongs

Inspect teeth, ensuring all teeth are present

Volkmann Retractor

Crile Retractor

Proper Name: Crile Retractor

Type: Hand-held

Size: 4.5"

Tray Assembly Tips: Small retractors should go on top or side of tray

Surgical Use: Small incision retraction

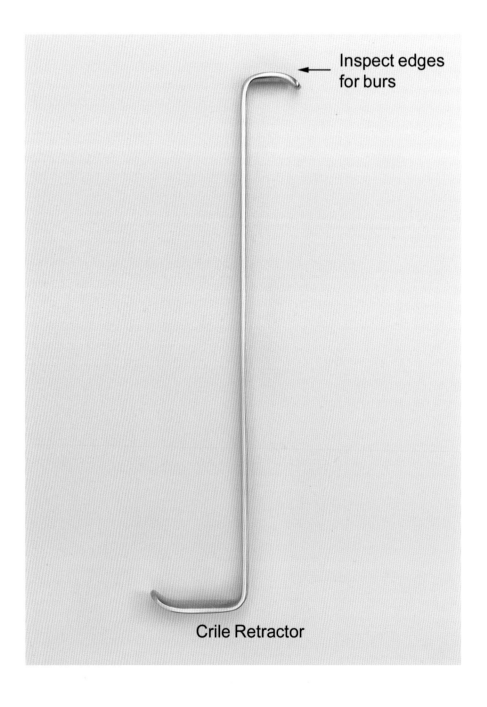

Inspect edges
for burs

Crile Retractor

Harrington Retractor

Proper Name: Harrington Retractor

Other Name: Sweetheart Retractor

Type: Hand-held

Size: Length: 12" - Width: 1", 1.5", and 2.5"

Tray Assembly Tips: Large retractors, such as the Harrington, should be placed in the bottom of the tray

Surgical Use: Deep tissue retraction

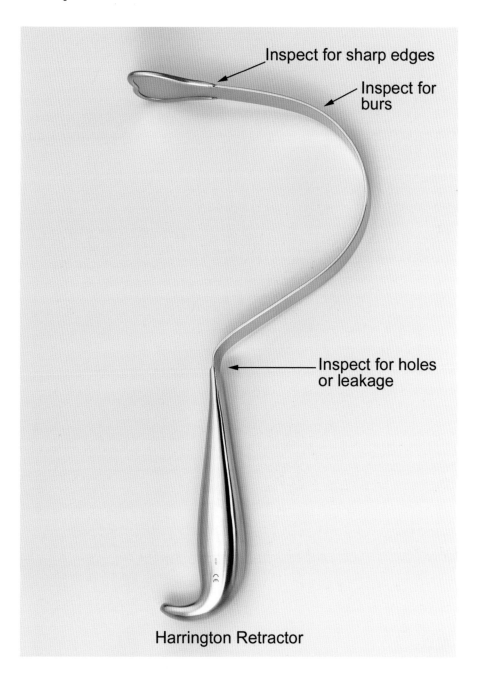

Harrington Retractor

Allison Lung Retractor

Proper name: Allison Lung Retractor

Length: 12.5", 2" wide blade

Tip Definition: Wire formed retractor blade

Tray Assemble Tips: Do not allow other instruments to get caught in metal wiring

Surgical Use: Retract and manipulate lungs

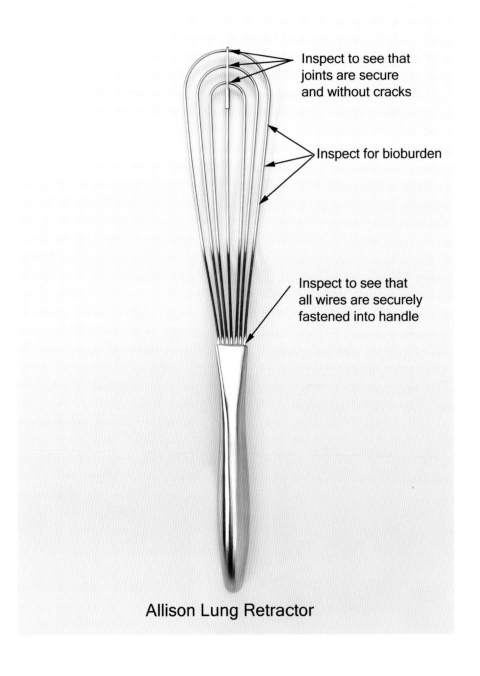

Inspect to see that joints are secure and without cracks

Inspect for bioburden

Inspect to see that all wires are securely fastened into handle

Allison Lung Retractor

Davidson Scapula Retractor

Proper Name: Davidson Scapula Retractor

Length: 3" wide x 3" deep blade

Surgical Use: Retracts scapula

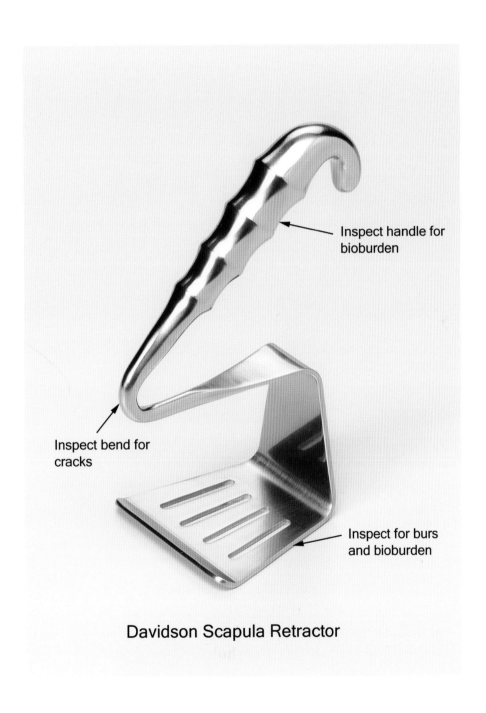

Inspect handle for bioburden

Inspect bend for cracks

Inspect for burs and bioburden

Davidson Scapula Retractor

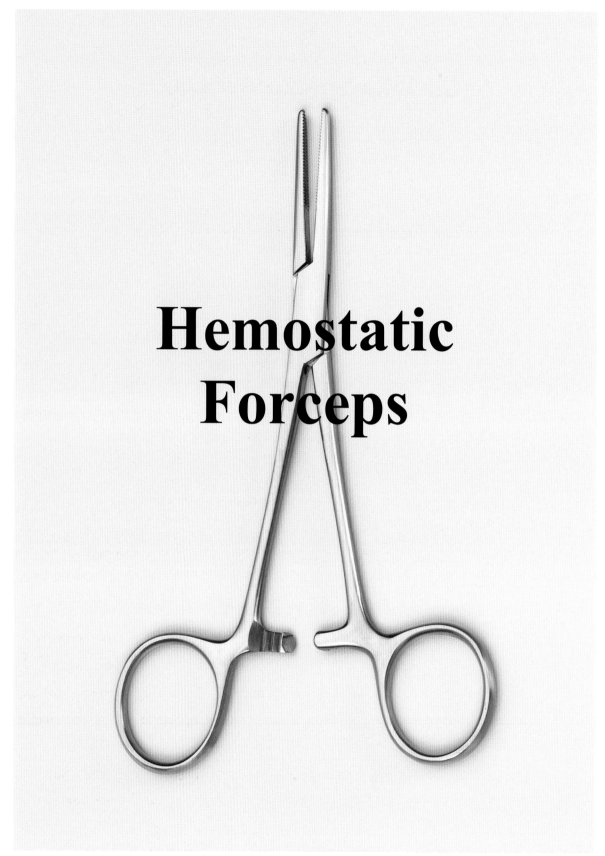

Hemostatic Forceps

Hemostats – primarily used to control blood flow via occlusion. Also used to grasp or hold.

Facts about Hemostats

- Hemostats are designed to hold all ratchets
- Hemostats should never be used to clamp any type of tubing
- Hemostats crack in the box lock area
- Hemostat jaws should fit together and not overlap
- Hemostats should never be sterilized with ratchets clicked and/or engaged

Points of Inspection:

- **Tips:**

    Serrated Hemostatic Forceps: (i.e. Rochester Pean, Crile, Kelly) should meet equally with no overlay.

    Hemostatic Tissue Forceps: (i.e. Allis, Kocher) Teeth at tips should be present, straight, and interfit precisely. Inspect teeth for bioburden.
- **Jaws:** Inspect serrations for blood or bioburden.
- **Box Lock:** Inspect for cracks on both sides of hinged area. This is the most common place to find blood and baked on bioburden.
- **Ratchet:** Ratchets should be tested every time prior to tray assembly. To test, simply open and close the hemostat. This action should be smooth and the ratchet should hold on each engagement (click). To further test ratchet to determine if it is sprung, set hemostat on first ratchet. Once secured on first ratchet, tap both rings softly and evenly on a flat table. If hemostat does not remain closed on first ratchet or springs open while tapping, the hemostat is in need of repair.
- **Post-Operative Care:** Always separate rings completely by opening ratchets. Never allow blood and bioburden to dry onto hemostat. To prevent blood from drying onto instruments and within twenty minutes of post op, soak instruments in an enzymatic solution or place a moist towel saturated with water over the instruments.

Hartman Mosquito Forcep

Proper Name: Hartman Mosquito Forcep

Other Names: Baby Snaps, Baby Mosquito

Similar Instruments with Same Inspections: Packer, Providence, Lahey, Coller, Rankin, Heaney

Jaw Definitions: Fully serrated jaw

Length: 3.5"

Surgical Use: To clamp off smaller vessels that control the flow of blood

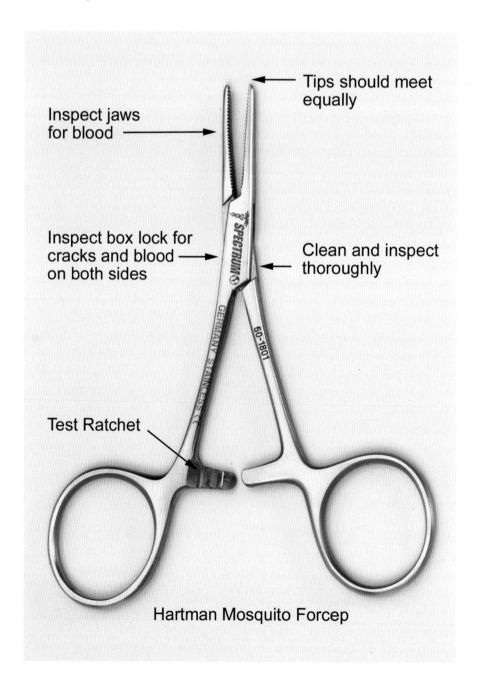

Tips should meet equally

Inspect jaws for blood

Inspect box lock for cracks and blood on both sides

Clean and inspect thoroughly

Test Ratchet

Hartman Mosquito Forcep

Halsted Mosquito Forcep

Proper Name: Halsted Mosquito Forcep

Other Names: Mosquitos, Stats, and Clamps

Jaw Definition: Fully serrated jaw

Length: 5"

Surgical Use: To clamp off smaller vessels that control the flow of blood

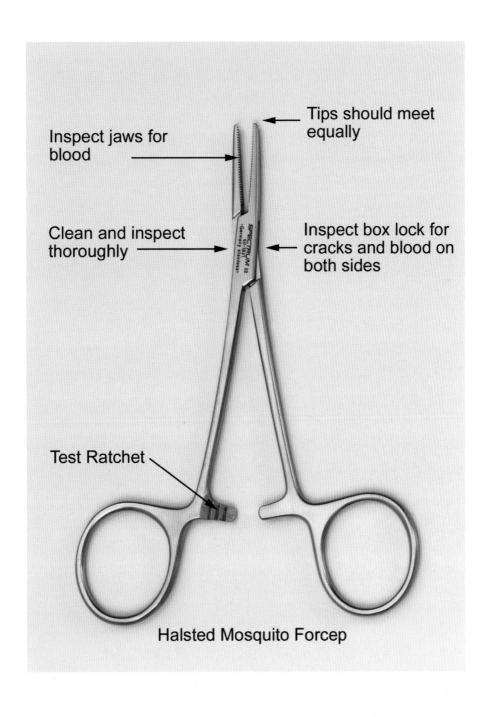

Tips should meet equally

Inspect jaws for blood

Clean and inspect thoroughly

Inspect box lock for cracks and blood on both sides

Test Ratchet

Halsted Mosquito Forcep

Kelly Hemostatic Forcep

Proper Name: Kelly Hemostatic Forcep

Other Names: Clamps, Snaps, Kellys

Jaw Definition: The Jaw is half serrated

Length: 5.5"

Surgical Use: To clamp off vessels that control the flow of blood

Kelly hemostats can also be used for blunt dissection

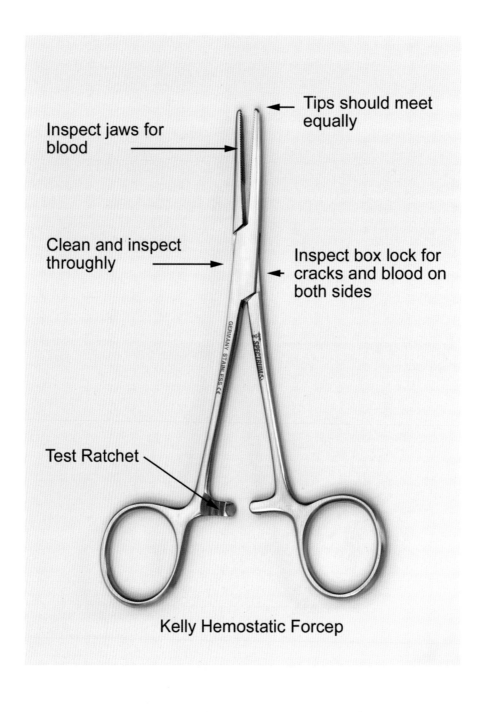

Tips should meet equally

Inspect jaws for blood

Clean and inspect throughly

Inspect box lock for cracks and blood on both sides

Test Ratchet

Kelly Hemostatic Forcep

Crile Hemostatic Forcep

Proper Name: Crile Hemostatic Forcep

Other Names: Often confused with Kelly Hemostat and Rochester Pean

Jaw Definition: The jaw is fully serrated

Length: 5.5"

Surgical Use: To clamp off vessels that control the flow of blood

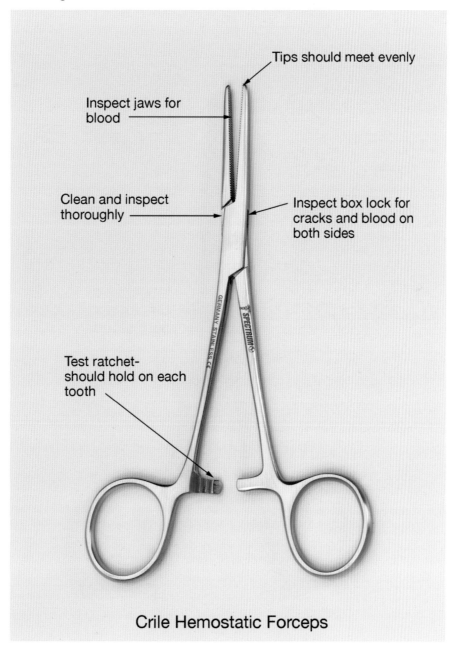

Crile Hemostatic Forceps

Rochester Pean Forcep

Proper Name: Rochester Pean Forcep

Other Names: Kelly, Big Hemostat, Pean

Jaw Definition: The Jaw is fully serrated

Length: 6.5" and 7.5" most common, up to 12"

Surgical Use: Used to occlude or clamp larger vessels to control bleeding

Note: Never use to clamp tubing

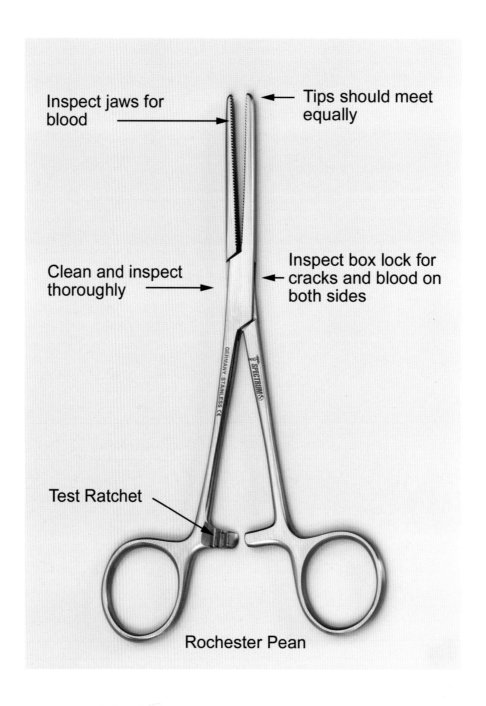

Inspect jaws for blood

Tips should meet equally

Clean and inspect thoroughly

Inspect box lock for cracks and blood on both sides

Test Ratchet

Rochester Pean

Allis Forcep

Proper Name: Allis Forcep

Similar Instruments with Same Inspections: Judd, Thomas

Jaw Definition: The distal tips have interlocking teeth. 3x4, 4x5, 5x6, 6x7

Length: 5.5" to 9"

Surgical Use: To hold and retract tissue, predominantly intestinal tissue

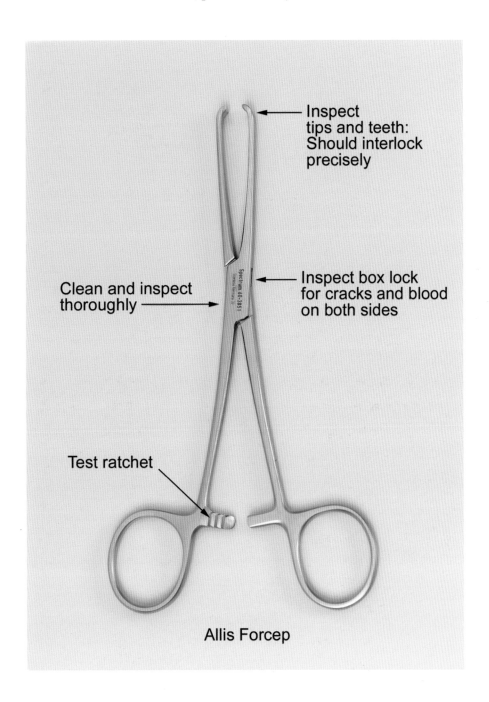

Inspect tips and teeth: Should interlock precisely

Inspect box lock for cracks and blood on both sides

Clean and inspect thoroughly

Test ratchet

Allis Forcep

Lahey Clamp

Proper Name: Lahey Clamp

Other Names: Tenaculum Forcep

Length: 6"

Jaw Definition: Has six interlocking teeth - check for missing teeth before sterilization

Surgical Use: To grasp tissue without crushing

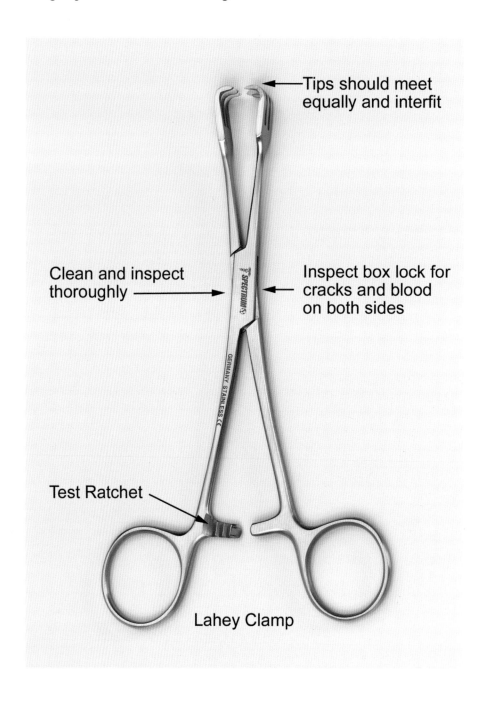

Tips should meet equally and interfit

Clean and inspect thoroughly

Inspect box lock for cracks and blood on both sides

Test Ratchet

Lahey Clamp

Babcock Forcep

Proper Name: Babcock Forcep

Other Names: Babcock Intestinal Clamps

Jaw Definition: Small, open half-circles with a horizontal serrated bar

Tips: Cross bar should meet evenly - inspect horizontal serrations for bioburden

Length: 6.5", 8" and 9"

Tray Assembly Tips: When assembling, make sure forceps are not engaged

Surgical Use: To grasp tissue in abdominal procedures such as the stomach, appendix, and gallbladder

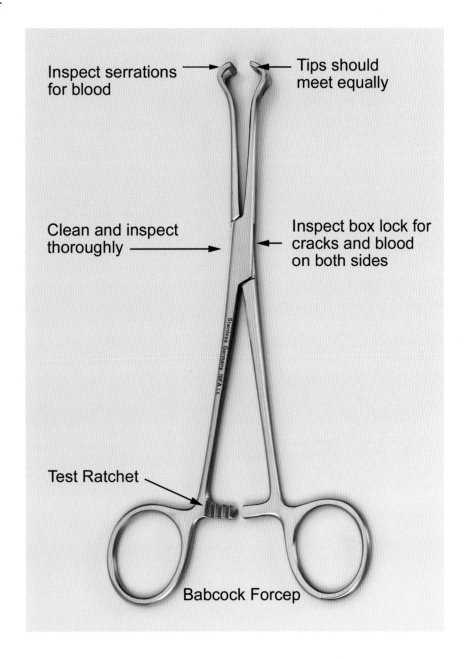

Inspect serrations for blood

Tips should meet equally

Clean and inspect thoroughly

Inspect box lock for cracks and blood on both sides

Test Ratchet

Babcock Forcep

Kocher Clamp

Proper Name: Kocher Clamp, Rochester (Oschner)

Other Names: Oschner, Hemostat with teeth

Length: 5" – 12"

Jaw Definition: 1x2 teeth at the tips - remainder of jaw has full length horizontal serrations

Tray Assembly Tips: When assembling, make sure ratchets are not engaged

Surgical Use: Grasping and holding muscle fascia

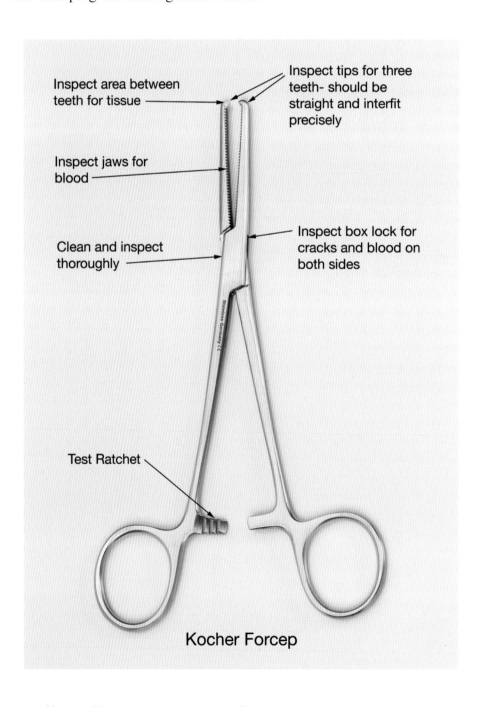

Kocher Forcep

Carmalt Forcep

Proper Name: Carmalt Forcep

Other Names: Rochester Carmalt, Stars and Stripes

Similar Instruments with Same Inspections: Bainbridge, Dennis, Allen

Jaw Definition: The jaw has longitudinal serrations and the tips have cross serrations

Length: 6.5" and 8", straight or curved

Surgical Use: For use on organs or tissues that are being removed such as the uterus

Note: This instrument is very crushing

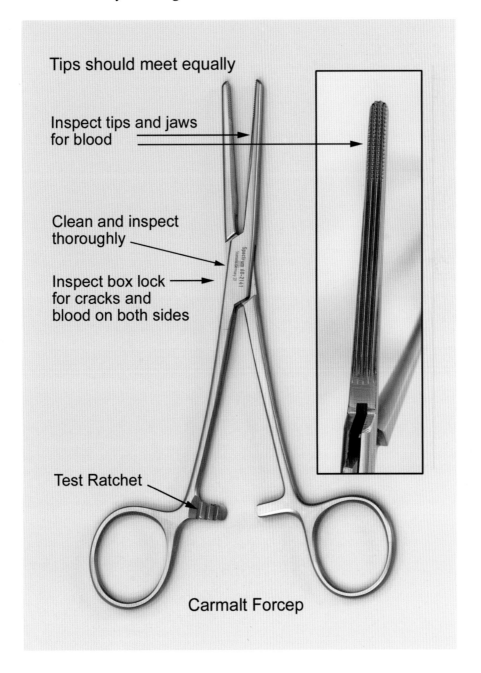

Tips should meet equally

Inspect tips and jaws for blood

Clean and inspect thoroughly

Inspect box lock for cracks and blood on both sides

Test Ratchet

Carmalt Forcep

Mixter Forcep

Proper Name: Mixter Forcep

Other Names: Right Angle, Debakey, Munion

Jaw Definition: Horizontal serrations the full length on jaw

Length: 6.5" – 12"

Surgical Use: Used for dissection of tissue in general and vascular surgery

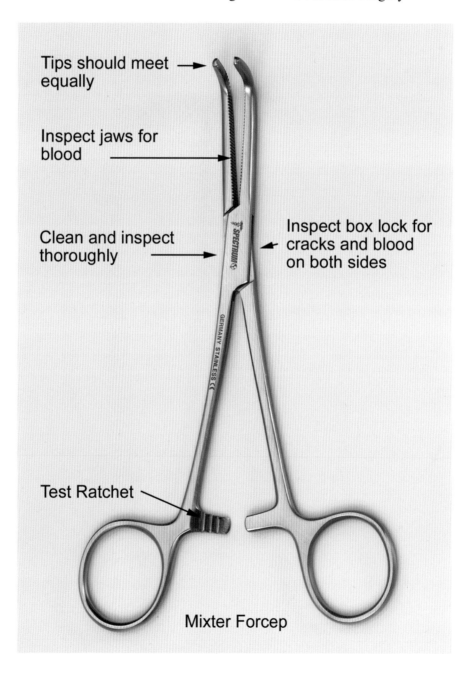

Tips should meet equally

Inspect jaws for blood

Clean and inspect thoroughly

Inspect box lock for cracks and blood on both sides

Test Ratchet

Mixter Forcep

Tonsil Forcep

- Schnidt
- Adson

Proper Name: Tonsil Forcep

Other Names: Schnidt, Sawtell, Open Ring Tonsil Forcep, Adson, White

Jaw Definition: Horizontal serrations on half of the length of the jaw

Length: 7.5"

Surgical Use: To clamp tonsils or other vessels and tissue

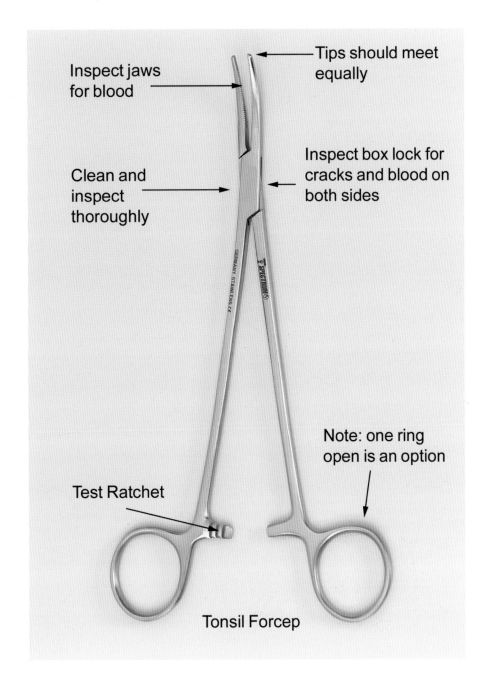

Inspect jaws for blood

Tips should meet equally

Clean and inspect thoroughly

Inspect box lock for cracks and blood on both sides

Note: one ring open is an option

Test Ratchet

Tonsil Forcep

Foerster Sponge Forcep

Proper Name: Foerster Sponge Forcep

Other Names: Sponge Stick, Sponge Clamp, Sponge Bob, Ring Forcep, Swab Stick

Jaw Definition: Oval tips with serrations

Length: 7.5" or 9.5"

Surgical Use: Holds sponges during preparation prior to incision

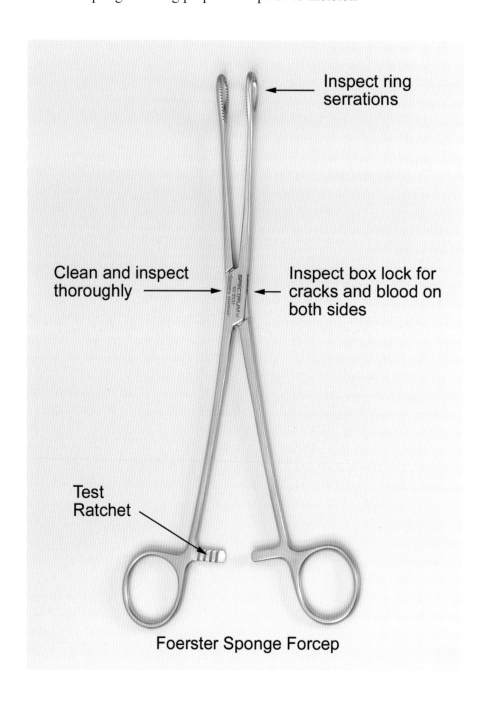

Foerster Sponge Forcep

Backhaus Towel Clamp

Proper Name: Backhaus Towel Clamp

Other Names: Towel Clamp, Towel Forcep

Jaw Definition: Jaws form a half circled point that overlaps when the sharp points meet

Length: 3.5" or 5.5"

Tips:

- Sharp points should be straight and overlap precisely when closing ratchet
- Be sure pointed tips are not bent or missing
- Tip protectors over sharp tips are a good practice to prevent accidental puncture

Box Lock:

- Inspect for cracks on both sides of hinged area
- This is also the most common place to find blood and baked on bioburden

Surgical Use: Secures sterile drapes and towels

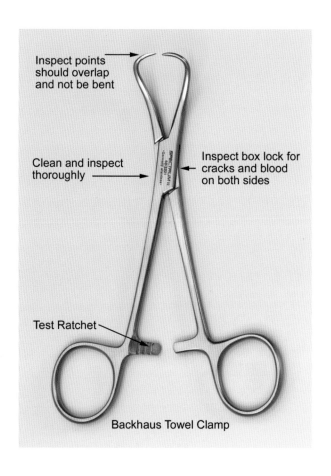

Backhaus Towel Clamp

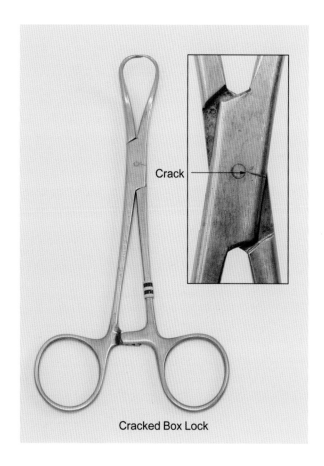

Cracked Box Lock

Jones Towel Forcep

Proper Name: Jones Towel Forcep

Other Names: Cross Action Towel Clamp

Similar Instruments with Same Inspection: None

Jaw Definition: Two pointed tips

Length: 2.5" and 3.5"

Surgical Use: For securing sterile drapes

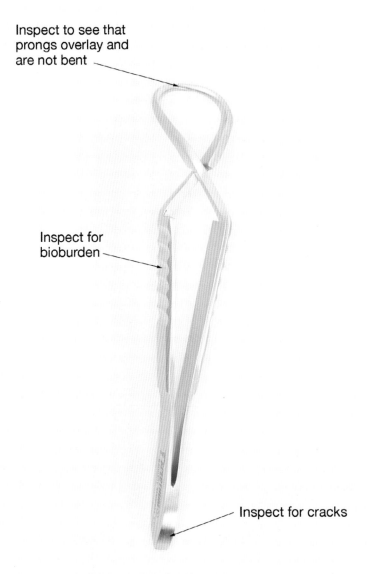

Inspect to see that prongs overlay and are not bent

Inspect for bioburden

Inspect for cracks

Jones Towel Forcep

Peers Towel Clamp

Proper Name: Peers Towel Clamp

Other Names: Non-Perforating Towel Clamp, Blunt Towel Clamp

Length: 5.5" and 6.5"

Jaw Definition:

- The distal jaws are rectangular and serrated
- Inspect rectangular jaw serrations for paper drape or prep solution

Tips: Should meet equally and flat

Surgical Use: To secure disposable/paper drapes without tearing or perforating. Extra large ratchets are to secure large amounts of drape

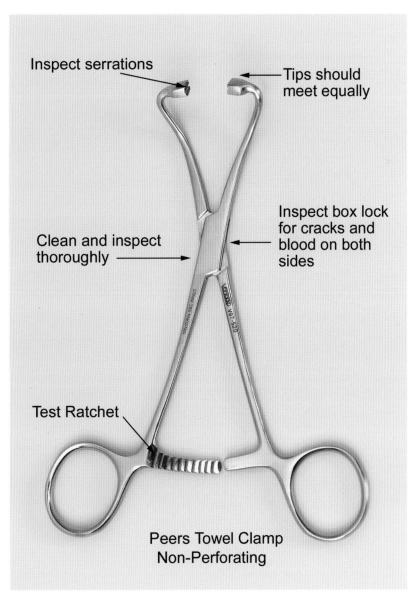

Inspect serrations

Tips should meet equally

Clean and inspect thoroughly

Inspect box lock for cracks and blood on both sides

Test Ratchet

Peers Towel Clamp
Non-Perforating

Tube Occluding Clamp

Proper Name: Tube Occluding Clamp

Other Names: Presbyterian, Vorse

Jaw Definition:

- Produced with either smooth jaws or lightly serrated jaws
- Jaws do not touch each other on this instrument

Length: 5", 6", 6.5", 7", 7.5", 8"

Surgical Use: Used to clamp off chest tubes, perfusionist tubing, and any other tube that needs a mechanical device to restrict flow

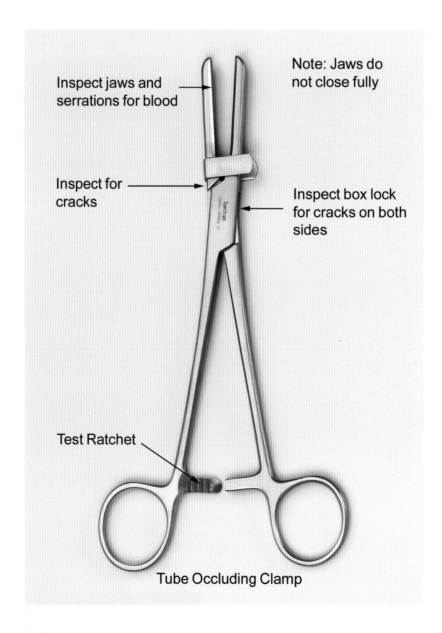

Inspect jaws and serrations for blood

Note: Jaws do not close fully

Inspect for cracks

Inspect box lock for cracks on both sides

Test Ratchet

Tube Occluding Clamp

Ferguson Angiotribe

Proper Name: Ferguson Angiotribe

Other Names: Angiotribe

Similar Instruments with Same Inspection: Hemostats

Jaw Definition: Cross serrated jaw with slotted groove the entire length of jaw

Length: 6.5" and 7.5"

Surgical Use: To clamp and crush removable tissue and organs

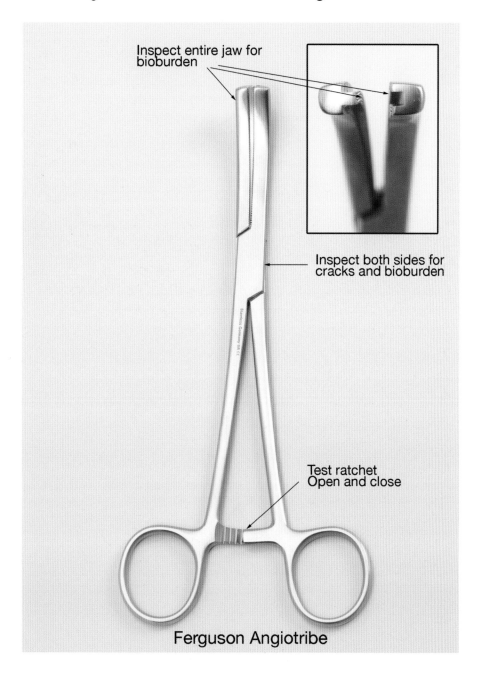

Inspect entire jaw for bioburden

Inspect both sides for cracks and bioburden

Test ratchet Open and close

Ferguson Angiotribe

Doyen Forcep

Proper Name: Doyen Forcep

Other Names: Intestinal Forcep

Similar Instruments with Same Inspection: Dennis Clamp, Scudder Forcep, Mayo-Robson Forcep

Jaw Definition: Long jaws with longitudinal serrations

Length: 9"

Surgical Use: Clamping intestinal tissue

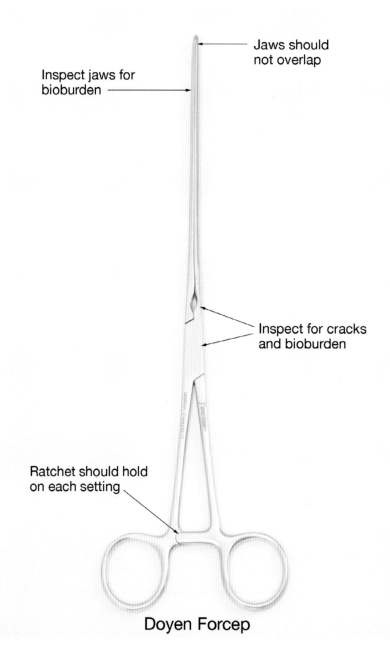

Jaws should
not overlap

Inspect jaws for
bioburden

Inspect for cracks
and bioburden

Ratchet should hold
on each setting

Doyen Forcep

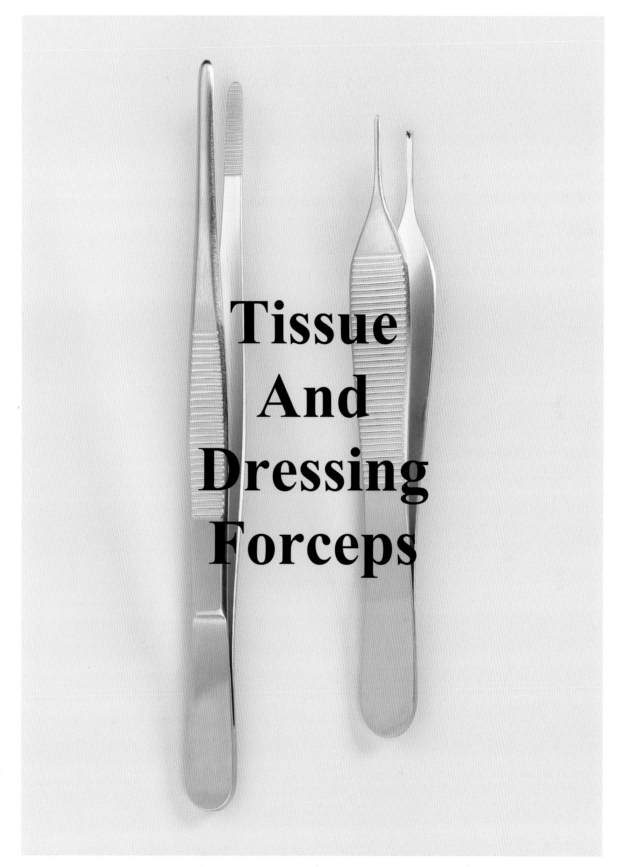

Tissue And Dressing Forceps

Tissue and Dressing Forceps – primarily used to manipulate, grasp, and hold tissue. Tissue forceps have teeth and dressing forceps do not.

Facts about Tissue and Dressing Forceps

- Opening and closing tension on a forcep does change with use
- Teeth will break off tissue forceps
- All teeth on tissue forceps should interfit
- Tissue and Dressing Forceps all crack at the proximal end
- Tissue and Dressing Forceps should not "click" and should not "stick" when testing

Points of Inspection

- **Tips:** Inspect tips to make sure there is no overlay and that tips meet evenly
- **Distal Serrations:** Inspect serrations for blood or baked on debris
- **Proximal End:** Inspect for cracks

Post Operative Care

Never allow blood and bioburden to dry onto clamp. To prevent blood from drying onto instruments and within twenty minutes of post-op, soak instruments in an enzymatic solution or place a moist towel saturated with water over the instruments.

Dressing Forcep

Proper Name: Dressing Forcep

Other Names: Thumb Forcep, Smooth Forcep, and Plain Forcep

Length: 4" to 12"

Tip Definition: Rounded tips with horizontal serrations

Cleaning Instructions: Follow standard decontamination procedures, followed by terminal sterilization procedures

Surgical Use: To pack and manipulate sponges and dressings - can also be used to handle and manipulate tissue

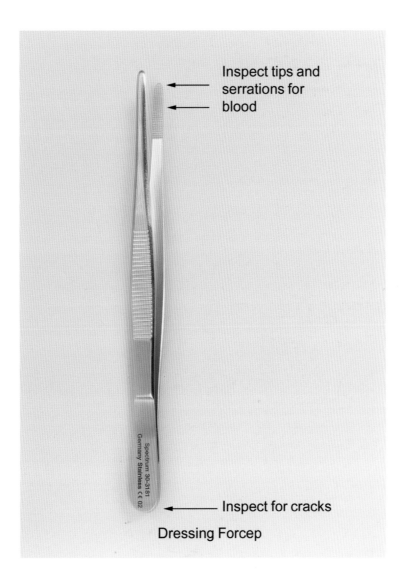

Inspect tips and serrations for blood

Inspect for cracks

Dressing Forcep

Tissue Forcep

Proper Name: Tissue Forcep

Other Names: Thumb Forcep with Teeth, Rat Tooth

Length: 4" to 12"

Tip Definition: Interlocking teeth of the same size: 1x2, 2x3, 3x4, 4x5

Cleaning Instructions: Follow standard decontamination procedures, followed by terminal sterilization procedures

Surgical Use: Manipulating and holding tissue during suturing

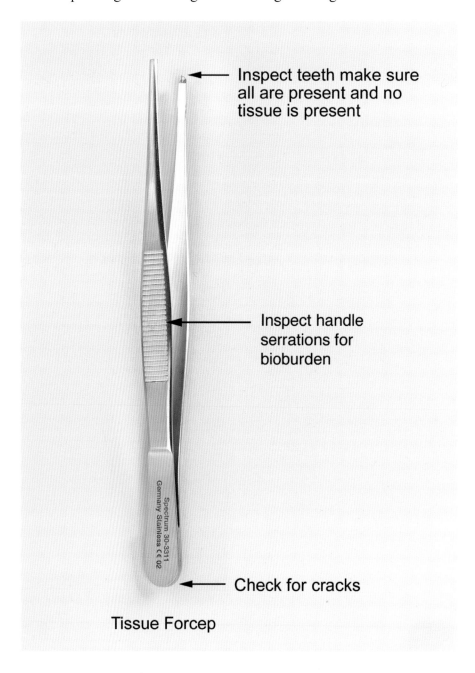

Inspect teeth make sure all are present and no tissue is present

Inspect handle serrations for bioburden

Check for cracks

Tissue Forcep

Adson Dressing Forcep

Proper Name: Adson Dressing Forcep

Other Names: Adson Smooth, Adson Plain

Length: 4.75"

Tip Definition: Rounded tips with serrations

Surgical Use: Manipulation of tissue during surgery

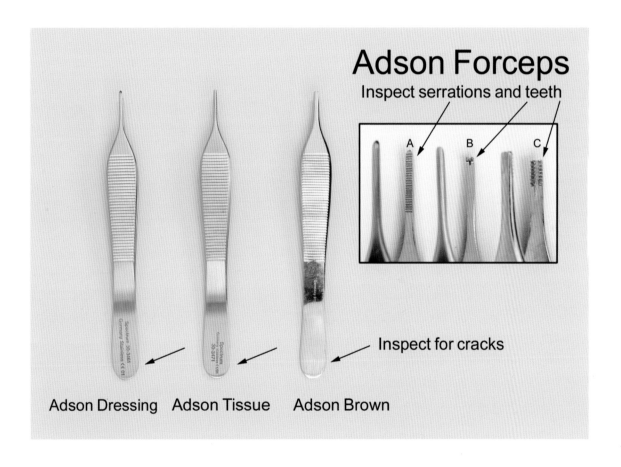

Adson Dressing   Adson Tissue   Adson Brown

Adson Tissue Forcep

Proper Name: Adson Tissue Forcep

Other Names: Adson with Teeth, Adson Rat Tooth

Length: 4.75"

Tip Definition: Three interlocking teeth of the same size

Surgical Use: Manipulation of tissue

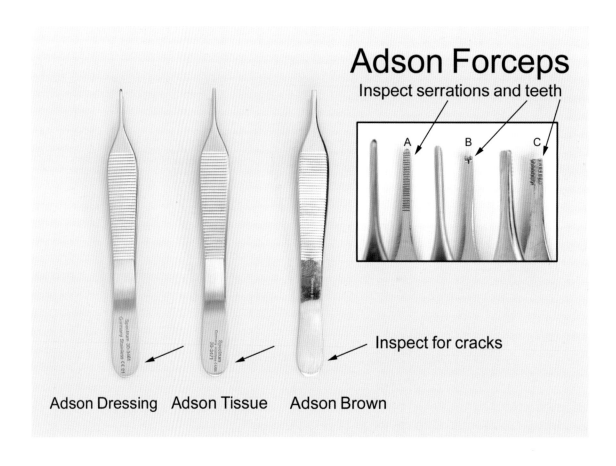

Brown Adson Forcep

Proper Name: Brown Adson Forcep

Other Names: Adson Brown, Multi-Tooth

Length: 4.75"

Tip Definition: Two rows of 7x7 interlocking teeth

Surgical Use: Less traumatic manipulation of tissue and used during suturing

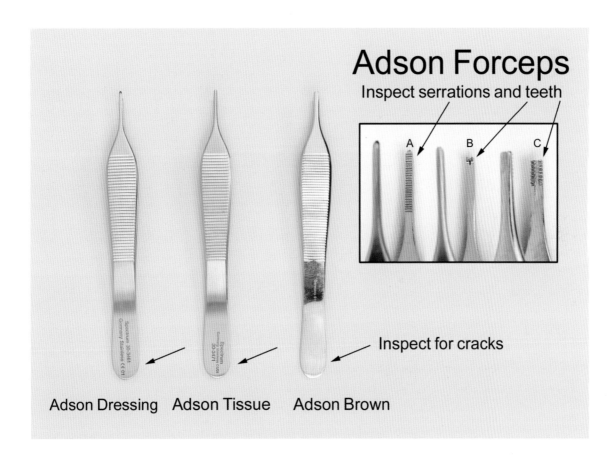

Adson Forceps
Inspect serrations and teeth

A   B   C

Inspect for cracks

Adson Dressing   Adson Tissue   Adson Brown

Debakey Tissue Forcep

Proper Name: Debakey Tissue Forcep

Other Names: Atraumatic Forcep, Debakeys, Vascular Forcep

Length: 6" – 11"

Jaw Width: 1.0mm, 1.5mm, 2.0mm, 2.5mm, 3.0mm

Tip Definition: Two rows of microscopic teeth that interfit along two slender jaws, ending with rounded distal tips

Spring Tension: This evaluation is very important on Debakey Forceps

The action of opening and closing the Debakey Forcep should be soft and easy - many times vascular forceps become "flattened" or spread open, which surgeons reject

Surgical Use: Less traumatic manipulation of tissue and used during suturing

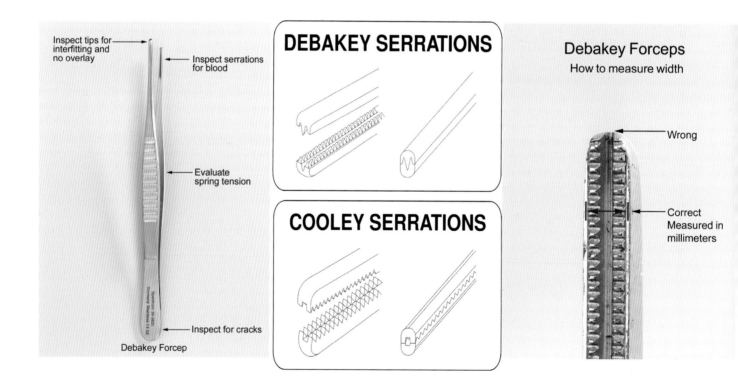

Russian Forcep

Proper Name: Russian Forcep

Other Names: Russians, Cat Paws

Length: 6", 8", 10", 12"

Tip Definition: Rounded distal tips with circular interlocking serrations with outer horizontal serrations

Surgical Use: Grasping tissue and organs

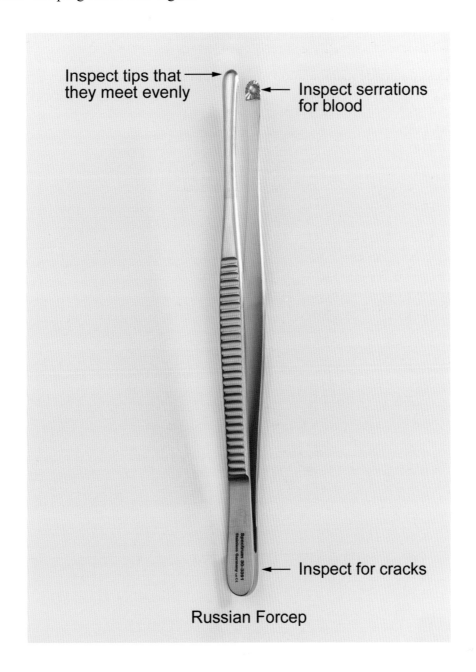

Inspect tips that they meet evenly

Inspect serrations for blood

Inspect for cracks

Russian Forcep

Ferris Smith Forcep

Proper Name: Ferris Smith Forcep

Other Name: Heavy Forcep

Length: 7"

Tip Definition: Large teeth followed by large serrations and teeth configuration: 1x2 or 2x3

Surgical Use: Heavy-duty tissue manipulation

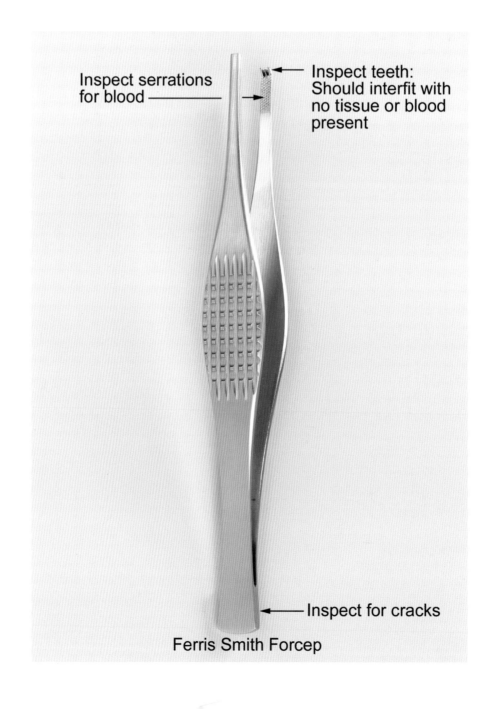

Inspect serrations for blood

Inspect teeth: Should interfit with no tissue or blood present

Inspect for cracks

Ferris Smith Forcep

Bonney Tissue Forcep

Proper Name: Bonney Tissue Forcep

Other Name: Large rat tooth

Length: 7"

Tip Definition: Large interfitting 1x2 or 2x3 teeth - behind teeth are serrations

Surgical Use: General and heavy suturing and manipulation

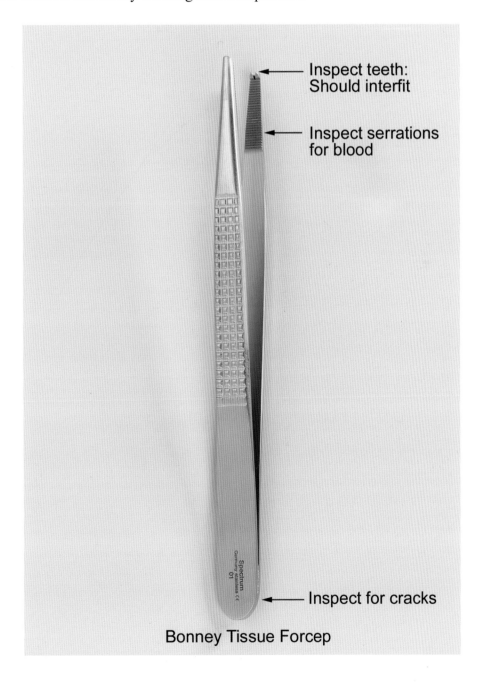

Inspect teeth:
Should interfit

Inspect serrations
for blood

Inspect for cracks

Bonney Tissue Forcep

Inspecting Gold Handled Tissue and Dressing Forceps

A gold-plated proximal end on tissue or dressing forceps indicates that the working portion of instrument contains tungsten carbide inserts. Tungsten carbide inserts must be inspected for tread wear, cracks, and/or missing pieces. This distal tip inspection should be performed prior to tray assembly.

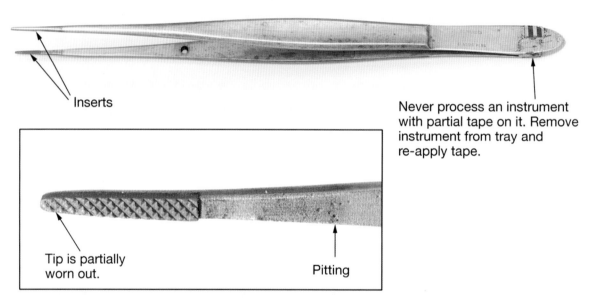

Inserts

Never process an instrument with partial tape on it. Remove instrument from tray and re-apply tape.

Tip is partially worn out.

Pitting

Damaged Potts-Smith Forcep

Potts-Smith Dressing Forcep

Proper Name: Potts-Smith Dressing Forcep

Other Names: Potts

Similar Instruments with Same Inspection: Dressing Forcep

Jaw Definition: Cross serrated jaws made from Tungsten Carbide or stainless steel

Length: 7", 8", and 9"

Surgical Use: To pick up and hold delicate tissue and fine suture

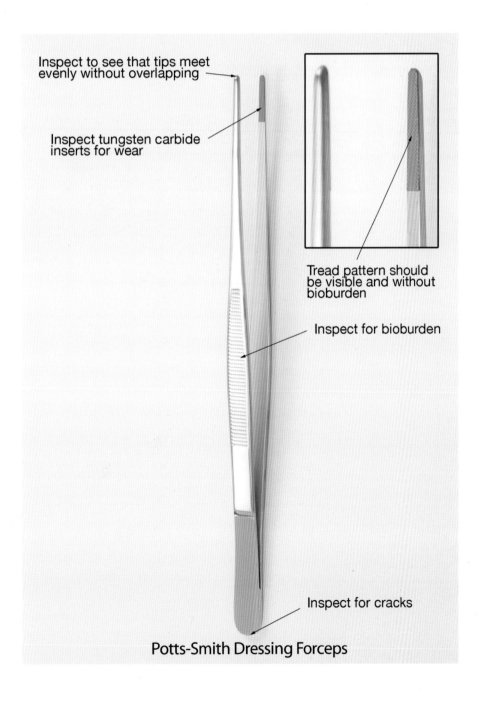

Inspect to see that tips meet evenly without overlapping

Inspect tungsten carbide inserts for wear

Tread pattern should be visible and without bioburden

Inspect for bioburden

Inspect for cracks

Potts-Smith Dressing Forceps

Adson Tissue Forcep with Suture Platform

Proper Name: Adson Tissue Forcep with Suture Platform

Other Names: Gold Adson

Similar Instruments With Same Inspection: Any other tissue forcep

Jaw Definition: 1x2 teeth with Tungsten Carbide pads set behind teeth

Length: 4.5" or 6"

Surgical Use: Tissue manipulation and the ability to grab suture needles

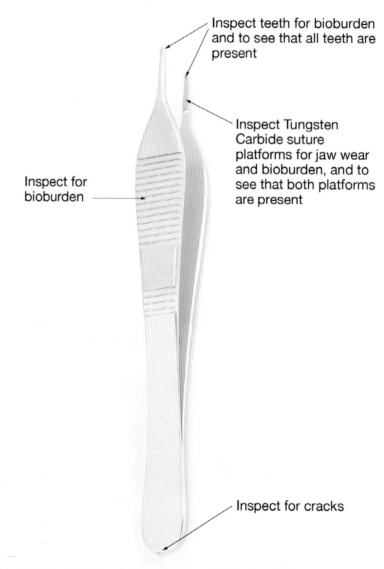

Inspect teeth for bioburden and to see that all teeth are present

Inspect Tungsten Carbide suture platforms for jaw wear and bioburden, and to see that both platforms are present

Inspect for bioburden

Inspect for cracks

Adson Tissue Forcep With Suture Platform

Singley Tissue Forcep

Proper Name: Singley Tissue Forcep

Other Names: Ring Forcep

Similar Instruments with Same Inspection: Tissue Forceps

Jaw Definition: Fenestrated and serrated jaw

Length: 9"

Surgical Use: To pick up and manipulate tissue

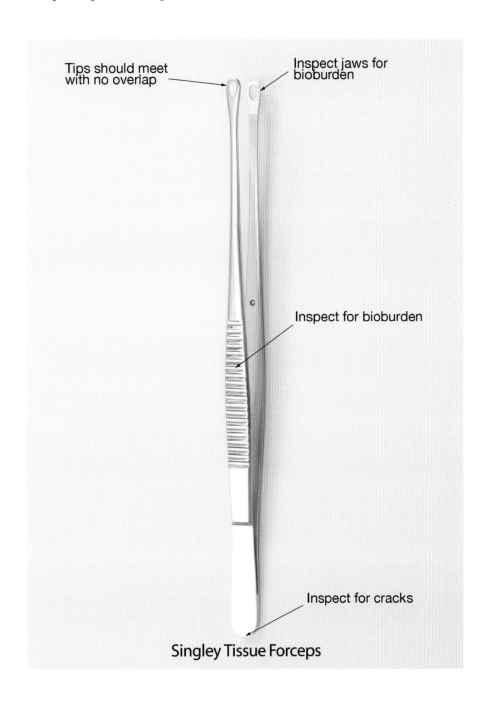

Singley Tissue Forceps

Jeweler Style Forcep (Style 3)

Proper Name: Jeweler Style Forcep (Style 3)

Other Names: Fine Pointed Forcep, Dumont Forcep, Swiss Forcep

Similar Instruments With Same Inspection: All forceps

Jaw Definition: Two very fine pointed tips

Length: 4.75"

Surgical Use: Fine tissue manipulation

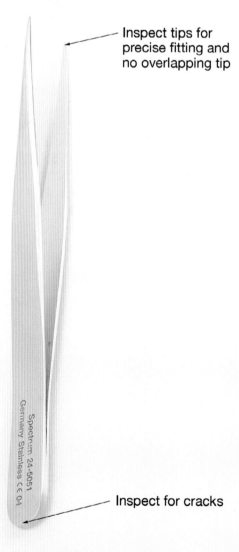

Inspect tips for precise fitting and no overlapping tip

Inspect for cracks

Jeweler Style Forcep

Bishop-Harmon Dressing Forcep

Proper Name: Bishop-Harmon Dressing Forcep

Other Names: None

Similar Instruments with Same Inspection: Graefe Forcep, Bonn Forcep, Lester Forcep

Jaw Definition: Two fine, serrated jaws

Length: 3.5"

Surgical Use: Fine tissue manipulation

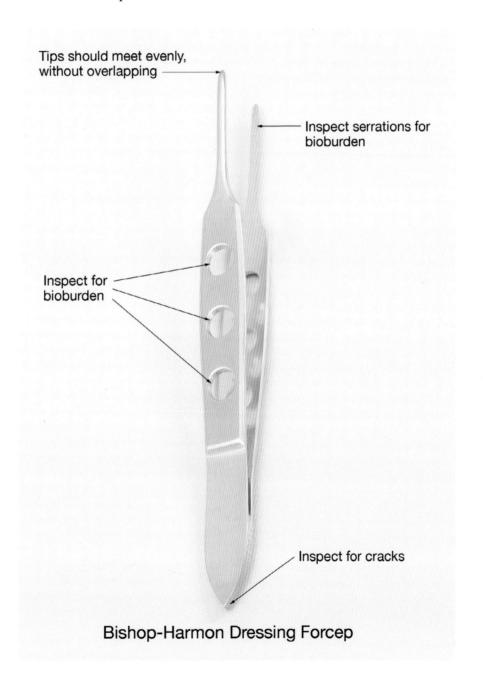

Tips should meet evenly, without overlapping

Inspect serrations for bioburden

Inspect for bioburden

Inspect for cracks

Bishop-Harmon Dressing Forcep

Jansen Dressing Forcep

Proper Name: Jansen Dressing Forcep

Other Names: Bayonet Forcep

Similar Instruments with Same Inspection: Adson Forcep, Gruenwald Forcep

Length: 6.25"

Surgical Use: Dressing and packing manipulation

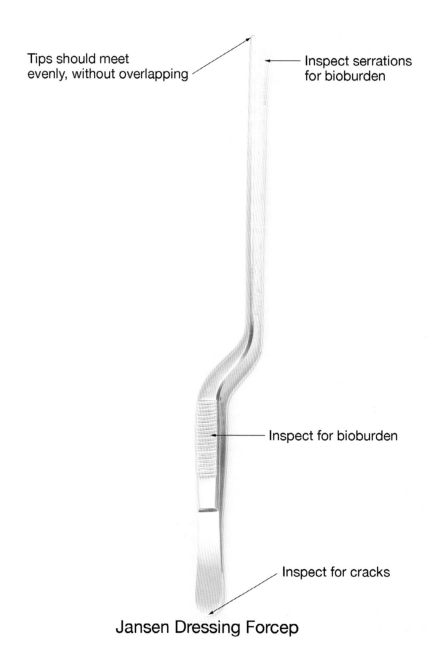

Tips should meet evenly, without overlapping

Inspect serrations for bioburden

Inspect for bioburden

Inspect for cracks

Jansen Dressing Forcep

- Bayonet.

Lucae Forcep

Proper Name: Lucae Forcep

Other Names: Bayonet Forcep

Similar Instruments with Same Inspection: Jansen, Gruenwald, Adson

Jaw Definition: Serrated jaws

Length: 5.5", 6.25", 8.25"

Surgical Use: For manipulating sponges and packing material during ear and nasal procedures

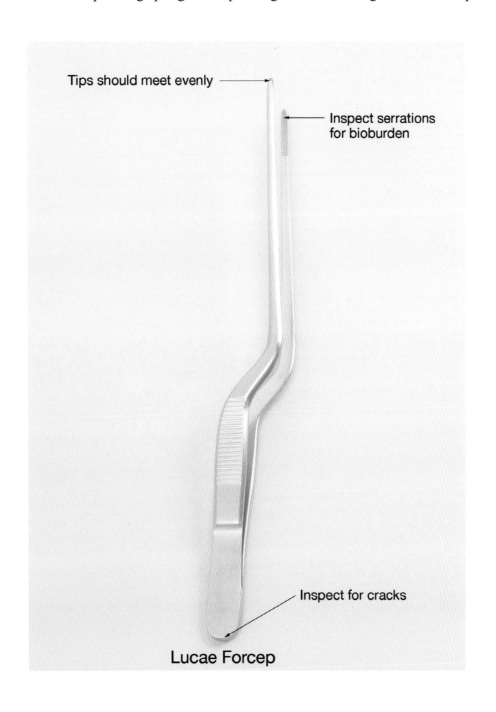

Tips should meet evenly

Inspect serrations for bioburden

Inspect for cracks

Lucae Forcep

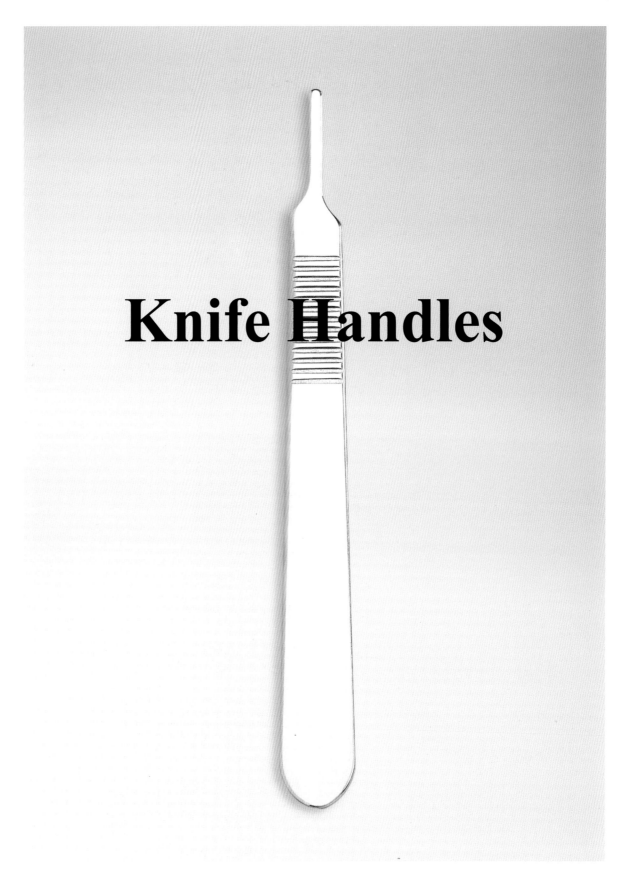

Knife Handles

Knife Handles – used to hold disposable scalpel blades of various shapes and sizes.

#3 Knife Handle

Proper Name: #3 Knife Handle

Other Name: Bard Parker #3

Size: 5"

Blades that fit: 10, 11, 12, 12B, 15, 15C

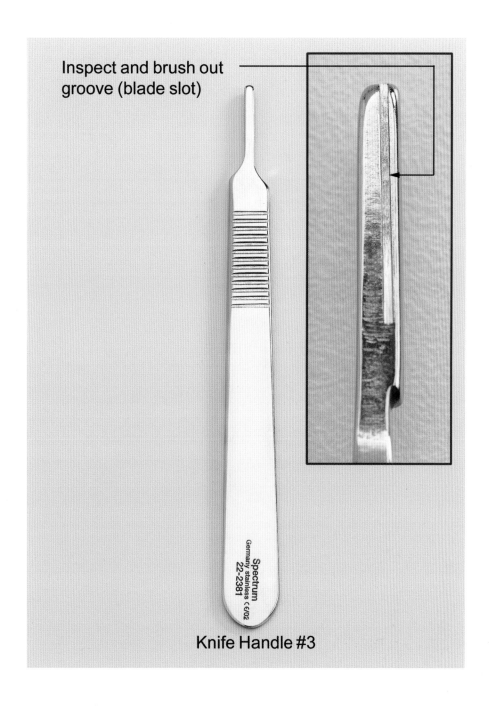

Inspect and brush out groove (blade slot)

Knife Handle #3

#3 Long Knife Handle

Proper Name: #3 Long Knife Handle

Size: 8"

Blades That Fit: 10, 11, 12, 12B, 15, 15C

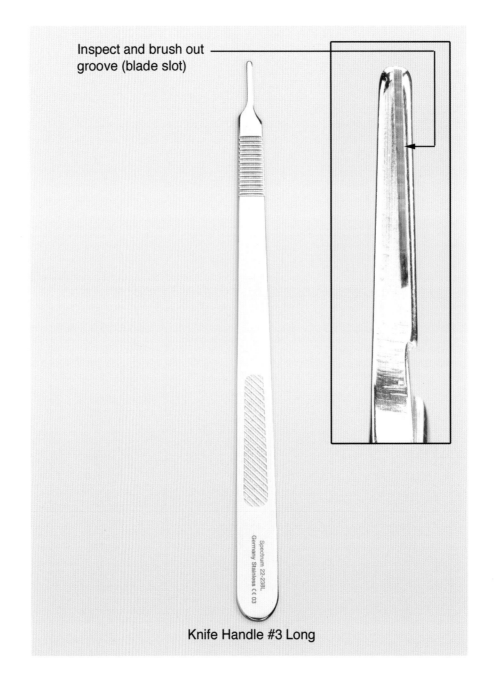

Inspect and brush out groove (blade slot)

Knife Handle #3 Long

#4 Knife Handle

Proper Name: #4 Knife Handle

Size: 5"

Blades that fit: 20, 21, 22, 23

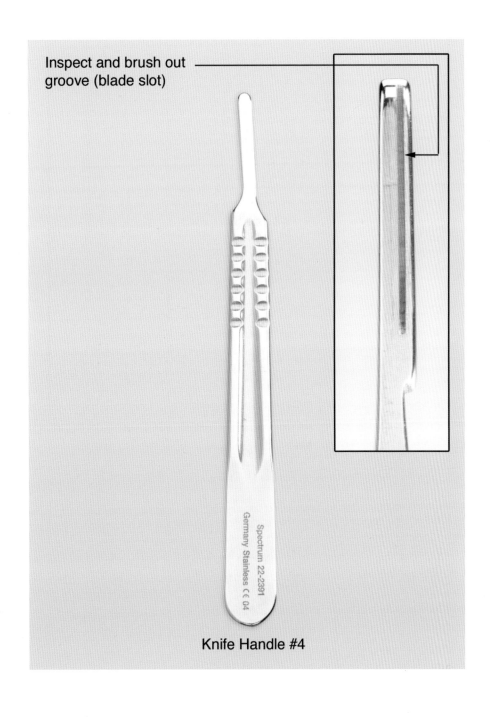

Inspect and brush out groove (blade slot)

Knife Handle #4

#7 Knife Handle

Proper Name: #7 Knife Handle

Size: 6.5"

Blades that fit: 10, 11, 12, 12B, 15, 15C

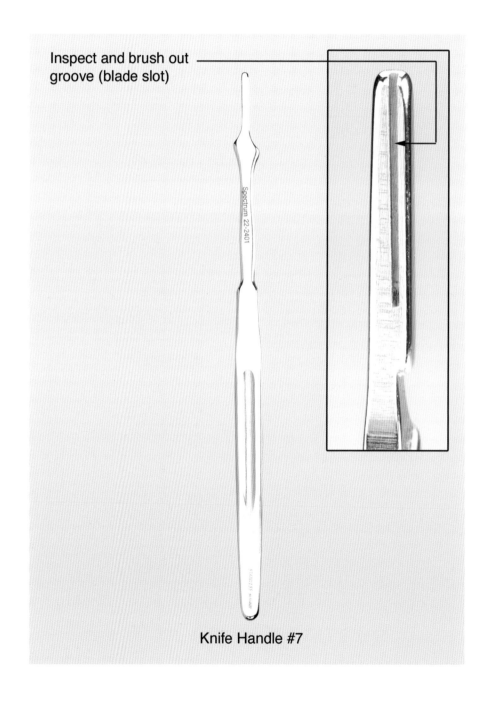

Inspect and brush out groove (blade slot)

Knife Handle #7

Micro Blade Handles

Proper Name: Micro Blade Handles

Other Name: Beaver Handle, Specialty Handle

Size: 4" and 5.5"

Blades that fit: 6100, 6200, 6400, 6700, 67MIS

Points of Inspection:

- **Distal tip:** Threaded blade fastening device must be present and smooth
- Thread tightening action

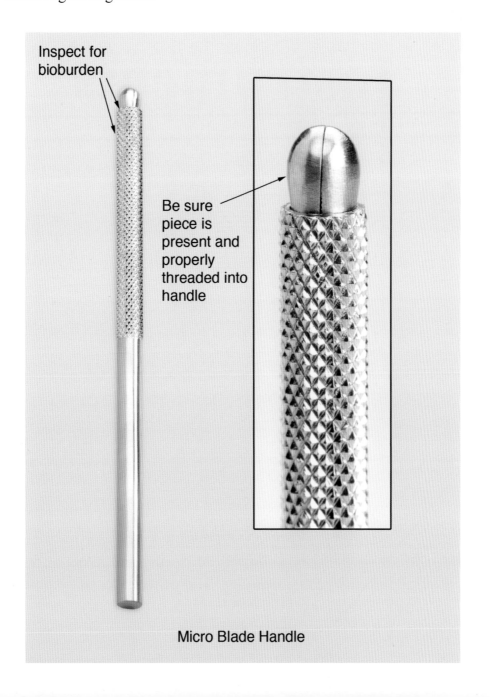

Inspect for bioburden

Be sure piece is present and properly threaded into handle

Micro Blade Handle

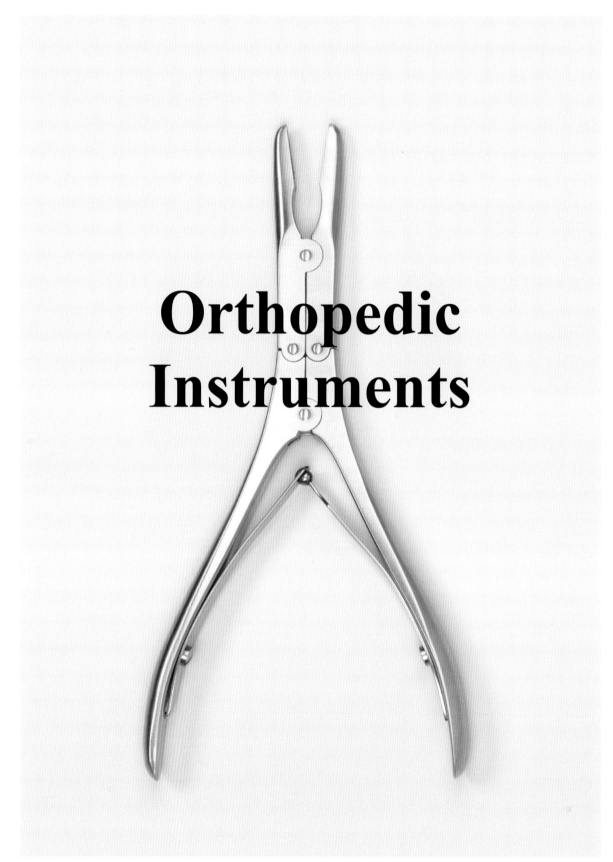

Orthopedic Instruments

Orthopedic Instruments – instruments used in surgical procedures that relate to the skeleton, its joints, muscles, and other related structures.

Gerzog Mallet

Proper Name: Gerzog Mallet

Similar Instrument with Same Inspections: Lucae

Length: 7.5", 8oz. Head

Tray Assembly Tip: Always place mallet in bottom of tray

Surgical Use: Use with osteotomes, gouges and chisels

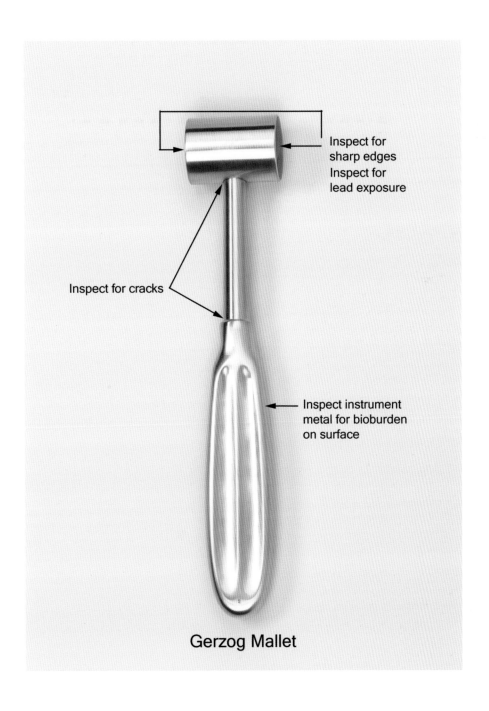

Inspect for sharp edges
Inspect for lead exposure

Inspect for cracks

Inspect instrument metal for bioburden on surface

Gerzog Mallet

Mead Mallet

Proper Name: Mead Mallet

Length: 7.5", 8 oz. head

Tip Definition: Nylon replaceable caps, used to reduce noise and prevent metal to metal damage

Tray Assemble Tips: Disassemble nylon caps for sterilization

Surgical Use: Use with chisels and osteotomes

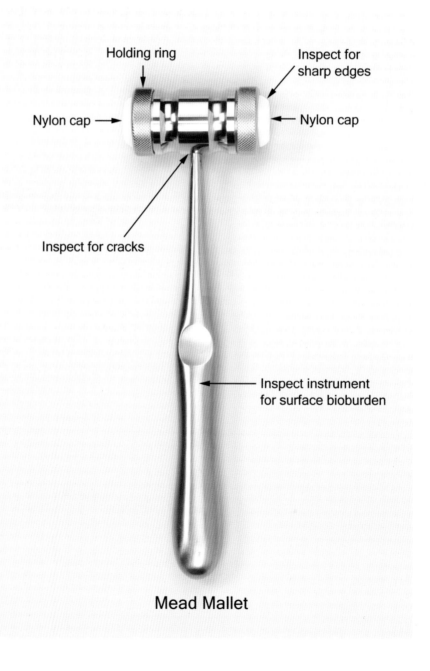

Mead Mallet

Evaluation of Osteotomes

As with most cutting devices, osteotomes must be routinely sharpened. Depending on case load and the number of osteotome sets, scheduled sharpening should be done four to six times per year. Over time, osteotomes get shorter due to the sharpening process as illustrated in the photo below. The most commonly used osteotome is usually the one that gets shortened the quickest. To determine if it is time to replace your osteotomes, simply measure it. Any osteotome that has been shortened by 1.5 inches or more from its original length should be replaced.

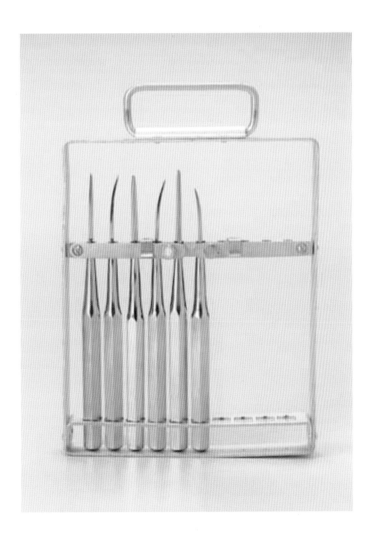

Lambotte Osteotome

Proper Name: Lambotte Osteotome

Similar Instrument with Same Inspections: None

Length: 9" straight and curved

Tip Definition: Sharpened on both sides

Width: .25", .5", .75", 1", 1.25", 1.5"

Criteria for Sharpness:

- See proper osteotome sharpening diagram
- Visually inspect with magnification for dented edges and corners
- Using plastic dowel rod, properly sharpened osteotome will shave off plastic

Surgical Use: Cutting and shaping bone

Tray Assemble Tips: Storage/sterilization racks as well as the use of tip protectors will protect cutting surface

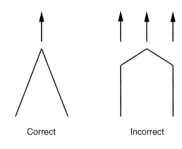

Correct   Incorrect

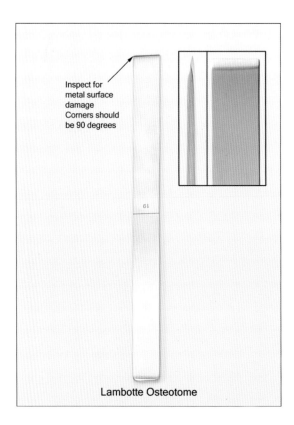

Inspect for metal surface damage Corners should be 90 degrees

Lambotte Osteotome

Hibbs Osteotome

Proper Name: Hibbs Osteotome

Length: 9", Straight or Curved

Tip Definition: Osteotome has an edge on both sides

Osteotome Width: 1/4", 3/8", 1/2", 5/8", 3/4", 7/8", 1",
1 1/8", 1 1/4", 1 1/2"

Points of Inspection:

- See proper osteotome sharpening diagram
- Visually inspect cutting edge with magnification for dented edges and corners
- Corners of osteotome should be 90 degree

Surgical Use: Cutting and shaping bone

Tray Assemble Tips: Sterilization trays or racks as well as the use of tip protectors will protect cutting surface

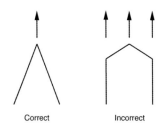

Correct   Incorrect

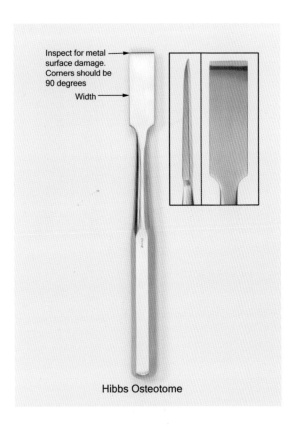

Inspect for metal surface damage. Corners should be 90 degrees

Width

Hibbs Osteotome

Hibbs Gouge

Proper Name: Hibbs Gouge

Length: 9" straight and curved

Similar Instrument with Same Inspections: None

Tip Definition: Round cutting surface

Gouge Width: 1/4", 3/8", 1/2", 5/8", 3/4", 7/8", 1", 1 1/8", 1 1/4", 1 1/2"

Criteria for Sharpness:

- Visually inspect with magnification to determine if surface damage is present
- Using plastic dowel rod, a properly sharpened gouge will shave off plastic

Surgical Use: Sharpening of bone

Tray Assemble Tips: Storage/sterilization racks as well as the use of tip protectors will protect cutting surface

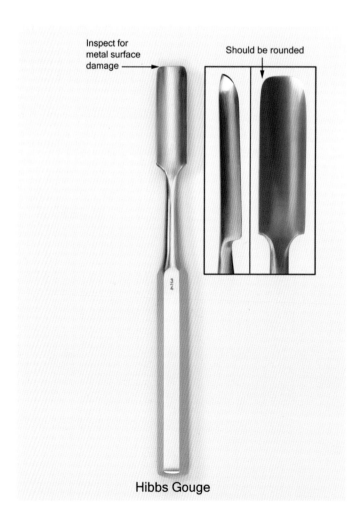

Hibbs Gouge

Hibbs Chisel

Proper Name: Hibbs Chisel

Length: 9" straight and curved

Tip Definition: A chisel is angled on one side

Width: 1/4", 3/8", 1/2", 5/8", 3/4", 7/8", 1", 1 1/8", 1 1/4", 1 1/2"

Points of Inspection:

- Inspect cutting edge for dented edges and corners
- Corner of chisel should be 90 degree

Criteria for Sharpness:

- Visually inspect with magnification to determine if surface damage is present
- Using dowel rod, a properly sharpened chisel will shave off plastic

Tray assemble tips: Sterilization trays or racks as well as the use of tip protectors will protect cutting surface

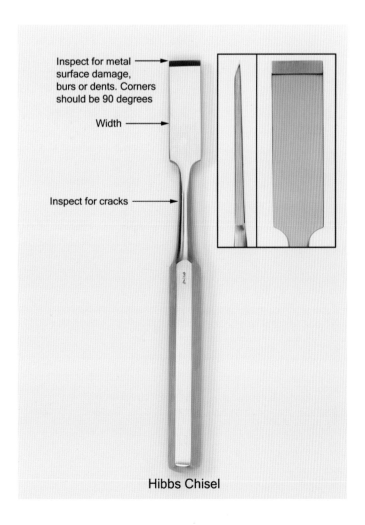

Hibbs Chisel

Hoke Osteotome

Proper Name: Hoke Osteotome

Length: 5.5"

Tip Definition: Osteotome width: 1/8", 3/16", 1/4", 5/16", 3/8", 1/2"

Points of Inspection:

- See proper osteotome sharpening diagram
- Inspect cutting edge for dented edges and corners
- Corners of osteotomes should be 90 degree

Criteria for Sharpness:

- Visually inspect with magnification to determine if surface damage is present
- Using plastic dowel rod, a properly sharpened osteotome will shave off plastic

Surgical Use: Cutting and shaving bone

Tray Assemble Tips: Tip protector will protect cutting edge of osteotome

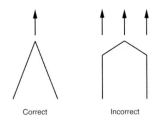

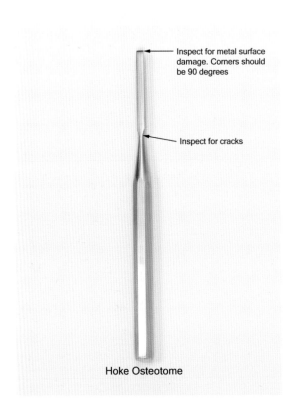

Hoke Osteotome

Key Elevator

Proper Name: Key Elevator

Other Names: Solid Handle Elevator

Similar Instruments With Same Inspection: Sayre Elevator, Chandler Elevator, Crego Elevator

Blade Definition: Semi-sharp, angled blade

Length: 7", 7.5", 8", 8.5"

Surgical Use: Used to separate muscle from bone

Sharpness Test Standard: Should scrape a plastic dowel rod

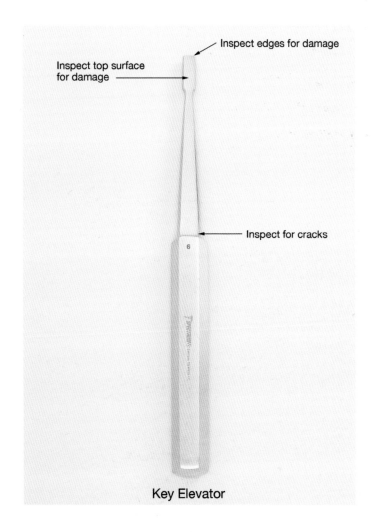

Inspect edges for damage

Inspect top surface for damage

Inspect for cracks

Key Elevator

Langenbeck Periosteal Elevator

Proper Name: Langenbeck Periosteal Elevator

Other Names: Joker, Cushing Joker

Similar Instruments With Same Inspection: Adson Elevator, Freer Elevator

Jaw Definition: Round, semi-sharp distal end

Length: 7.5"

Surgical Use: Used to separate muscle from bone

Sharpness Test Standard: Should scrape a plastic dowel rod

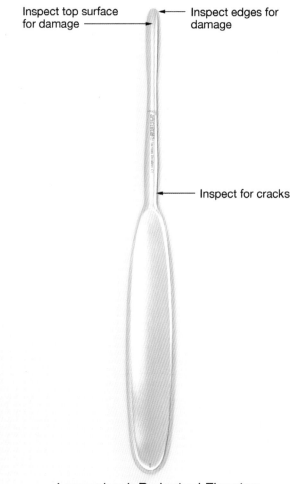

Inspect top surface for damage — Inspect edges for damage

Inspect for cracks

Langenbeck Periosteal Elevator

Lewin Bone Holding Forcep

Proper Name: Lewin Bone Holding Forcep

Similar Instruments with Same Inspections: Dingman

Length: 7"

Tip definition: Distal jaws have serrations

Tray Assemble Tips: Sterilize with ratchet open

Surgical Use: For reducing fractured bones and manipulation of bones

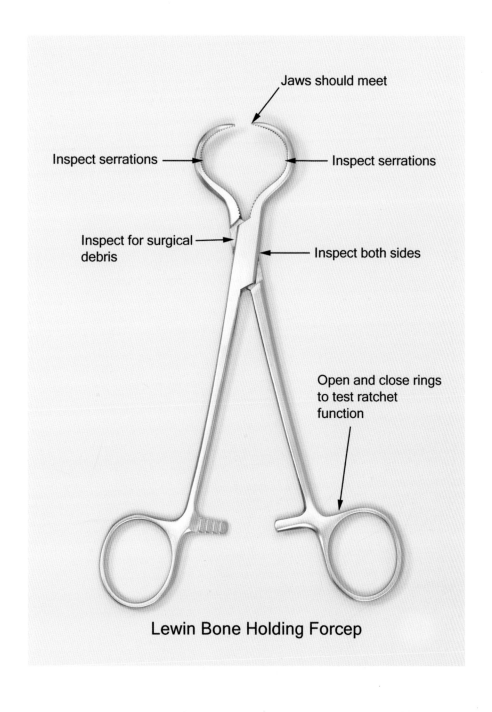

Jaws should meet

Inspect serrations

Inspect serrations

Inspect for surgical debris

Inspect both sides

Open and close rings to test ratchet function

Lewin Bone Holding Forcep

Lowman Bone Holding Clamp

Proper Name: Lowman Bone Holding Clamp

Length: 5", 7", 8", calibrated in .125"

Tip Definition:

- 1 x 2 prong jaws
- 5" clamp has .75" wide jaws
- 7" clamp has 1" wide jaws
- 8" clamp has 1.25" wide jaws

Surgical use: Used for reducing a long bone fracture

Tray Assemble Tips: Sterilize with jaws open

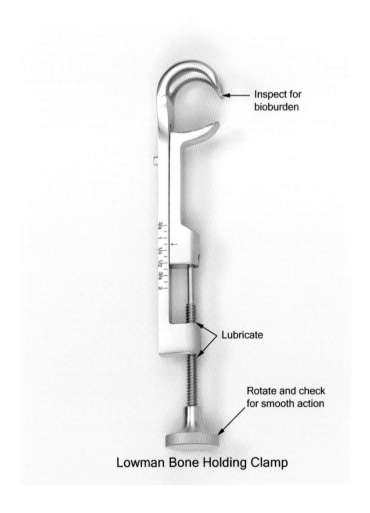

Lowman Bone Holding Clamp

Martin Cartilage Clamp

Proper Name: Martin Cartilage Clamp

Similar Instruments with Same Inspection: Hemostats

Length: 7" and 8"

Tip/Jaw Definition: Large and deep serrations

Surgical Use: Grasping of cartilage

Tray Assemble Tips: Assemble and sterilize with ratchet open

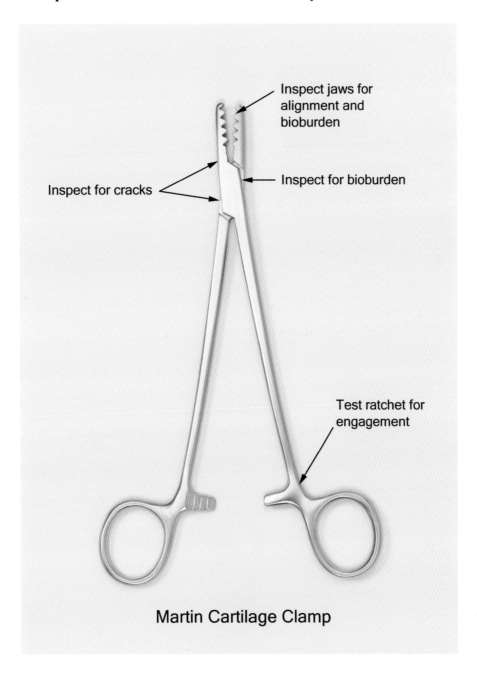

Inspect jaws for alignment and bioburden

Inspect for cracks

Inspect for bioburden

Test ratchet for engagement

Martin Cartilage Clamp

Periosteal Elevator

Proper Name: Periosteal Elevator

Similar Instruments With Same Inspection: Chandler, Sayre, Crego Key, Sedillot, Fomon

Jaw Definition: Softly rounded semi-sharp edges

Length: 7", 8", 9"

Surgical Use: For separating periosteum

Sharpness Test Standard: Should not be sharpened to a sharp edge - the edge of any elevator is a soft semi-sharp edge

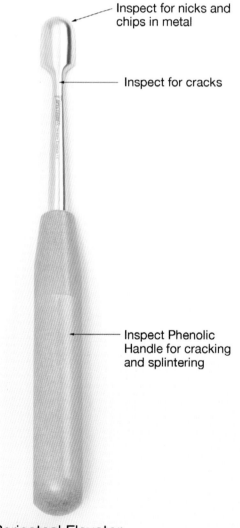

Inspect for nicks and chips in metal

Inspect for cracks

Inspect Phenolic Handle for cracking and splintering

Periosteal Elevator

Hohmann Retractor

Proper Name: Hohmann Retractor

Similar Instrument with Same Inspections: Smille, Blount

Length: 9.25" and 9.75" (6.25" defined as Mini Hohman)

Tip Definition: Various widths of blades: 6mm, 8mm, 10mm, 18mm, 25mm, 43mm, 70mm

Surgical Use: Retraction and leveraging joints

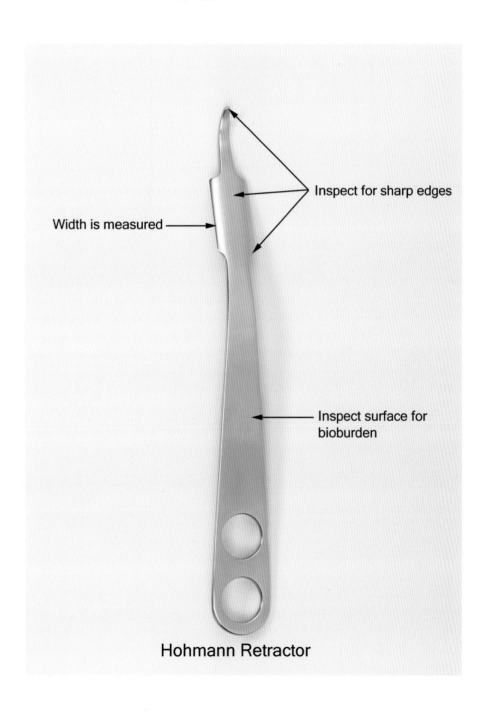

Hohmann Retractor

Jaw Inspection of Bone Cutters

Prior to tray assembly, the jaws of a bone cutter must be inspected. If any cutting edge surface damage is discovered, schedule the instrument immediately for repair and discontinue use.

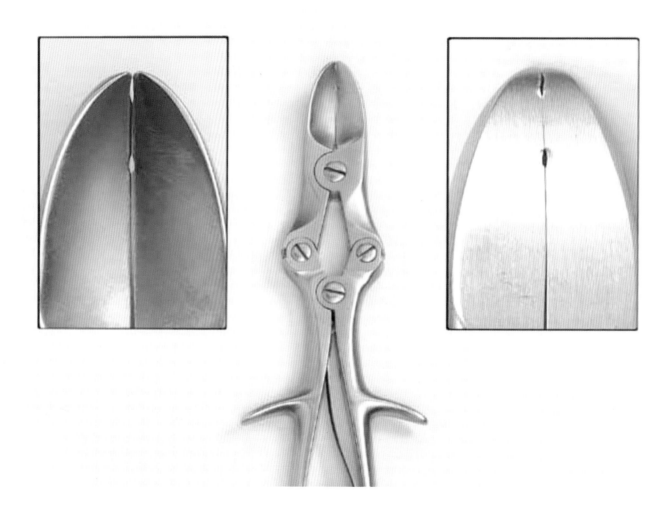

Ruskin Rongeur, Double Action

Proper Name: Ruskin Rongeur, Double Action

Similar Instruments with Same Inspections: Beyer, Leksell, Zaufel Stille

Length: 6" and 7.25"

Tip/Jaw Definition:

- Straight and curved jaws

- 3mm, 5mm, 7mm

- Jaw width referred to as bite

Criteria for sharpness: Should cut clean through an index card

Surgical use: Cutting and biting tissue or bone

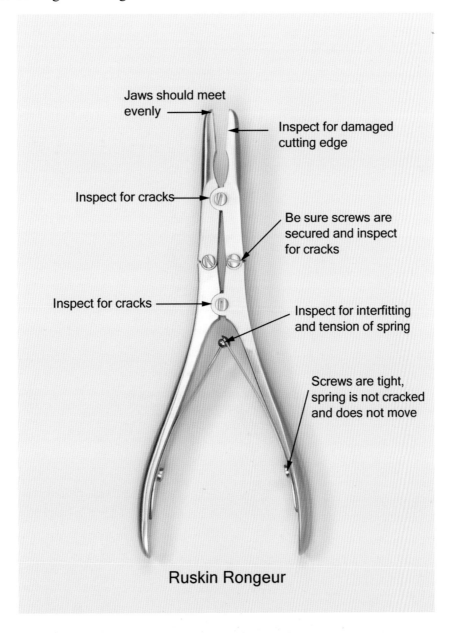

Ruskin Rongeur

Ruskin Bone Cutting Forcep

Proper Name: Ruskin Bone Cutting Forcep

Similar Instruments with Same Inspections: Kleinert-Kutz, Rowland

Length: 5.5" and 7.5"

Criteria for Sharpness: Should cut through an index card with front half of cutting blades

Surgical Use: Cutting and trimming bone and bone fragments

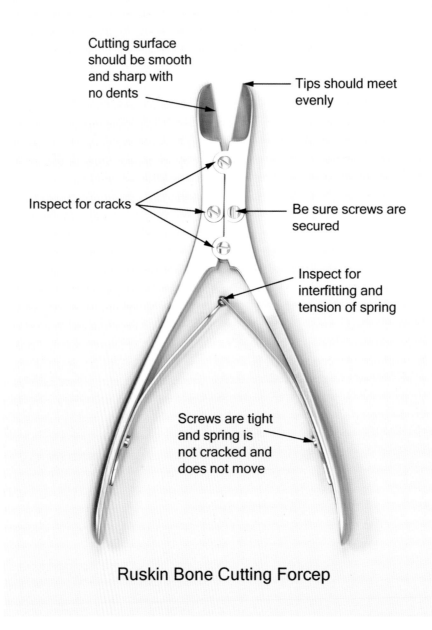

Cutting surface should be smooth and sharp with no dents

Tips should meet evenly

Inspect for cracks

Be sure screws are secured

Inspect for interfitting and tension of spring

Screws are tight and spring is not cracked and does not move

Ruskin Bone Cutting Forcep

Liston Amputation Knife

Proper Name: Liston Amputation Knife

Length: 11.75" and 13.75"

Tip Definition: Very sharp tip and blade

Criteria for sharpness: Plastic rod

Surgical use: Cutting of tissue, cartilage, and muscle

Caution: <u>SHARPS RISK</u>. Knife should always be in a protective sleeve when not in use

Tray Assemble Tips: Assemble in separate container or tray for sharps protection

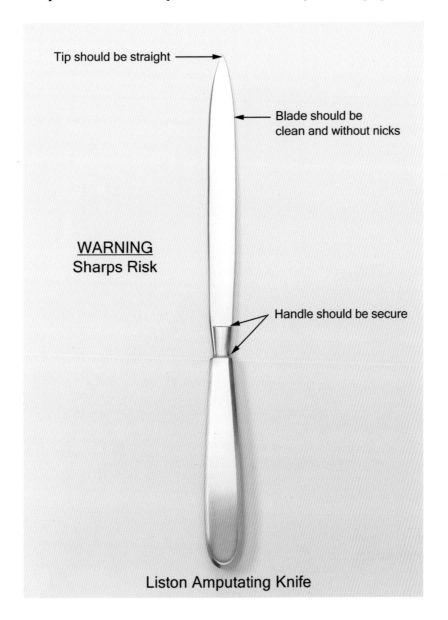

Tip should be straight

Blade should be
clean and without nicks

<u>WARNING</u>
Sharps Risk

Handle should be secure

Liston Amputating Knife

Pin Cutter (Flush)

Proper Name: Pin Cutter (Flush)

Other Names: Flush Cutting Pin Cutter, End Cutter

Similar Instruments With Same Inspection: Wire Cutter

Jaw Definition: Two sharp cutting edges

Length: 7.5", 8.5", 9.5"

Surgical Use: Cutting pins and wires near (flush) the surgical site

Sharpness Test Standard: Ability to cut maximum diameter pins and wires

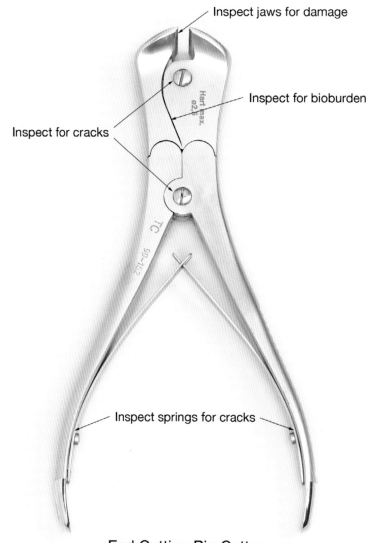

End Cutting Pin Cutter

Pin Cutter

Proper Name: Pin Cutter

Other Names: Side Cutting Pin Cutter, End Cutting

Similar Instruments With Same Inspection: Wire Cutter

Jaw Definition: Two sharp cutting, angled edges

Length: 7.5", 8.5", 9.5"

Surgical Use: Cutting pins and wires near the surgical site

Sharpness Test Standard: Ability to cut maximum diameter pins and wires

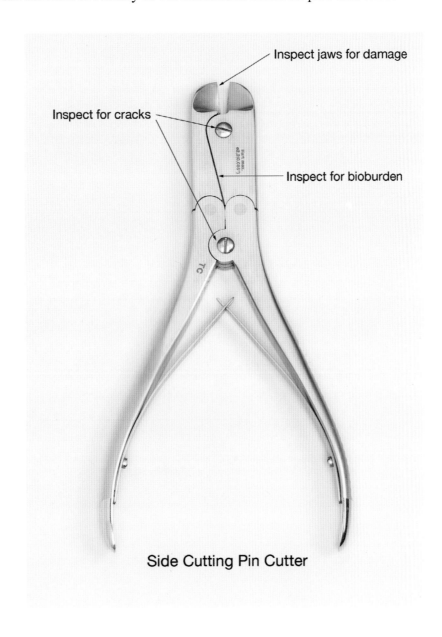

Side Cutting Pin Cutter

Cannulated Pin Cutter

Proper Name: Cannulated Pin Cutter

Other Names: End Cutter

Similar Instruments With Same Inspection: Pin and Wire Cutters

Jaw Definition: Two sharp cutting edges

Length: 7.5"

Surgical Use: Cutting small pins and wires

Sharpness Test Standard: Ability to cut 1/8" wire

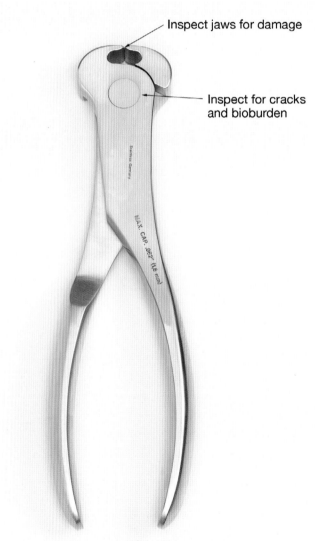

Inspect jaws for damage

Inspect for cracks
and bioburden

Cannulated Pin Cutter

Kern Bone Holding Forcep

Proper Name: Kern Bone Holding Forcep

Similar Instruments With Same Inspection: Lane, Lambotte, Farabeuf

Jaw Definition: Serrated jaws with two teeth on both sides

Length: 6" and 9.5"

Surgical Use: Manipulation of bones

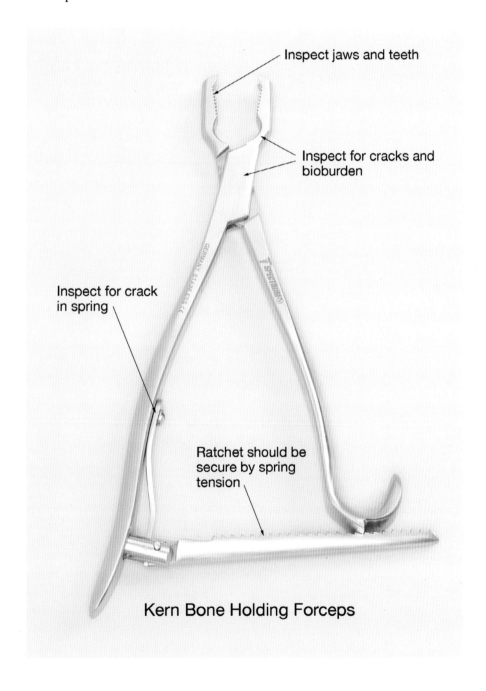

Inspect jaws and teeth

Inspect for cracks and bioburden

Inspect for crack in spring

Ratchet should be secure by spring tension

Kern Bone Holding Forceps

Doyen Elevator Rasp

Proper Name: Doyen Elevator Rasp

Similar Instruments with Same Inspections: None

Length: 7", adult and child

Tip Definition:

- Curved left and curved right
- Semi sharp cutting blades

Criteria for Sharpness: Semi sharp edge cuts into plastic dowel rod

Surgical use: Scrape tissue and cartilage from ribs

Tray Assemble Tips: Be sure left and right elevators are marked properly

Tray contains both a left and a right rasp

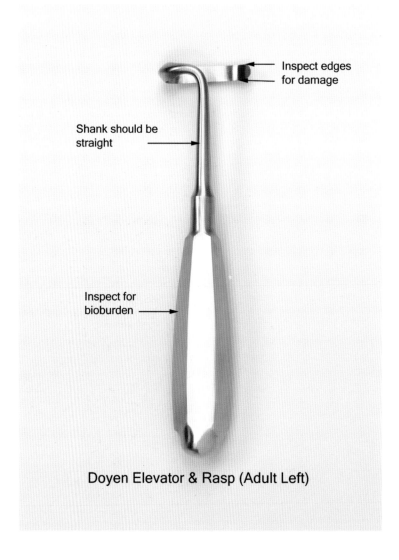

Inspect edges for damage

Shank should be straight

Inspect for bioburden

Doyen Elevator & Rasp (Adult Left)

Jaw Inspection of Cervical and Laminectomy Rongeurs

Prior to tray assembly, the distal tips of these neurological Rongeurs require a close inspection. Damaged or dented cutting surfaces significantly reduce the instrument's ability to cut. Both sides of the Rongeur should be inspected for damage and bioburden. If damaged, discontinue use.

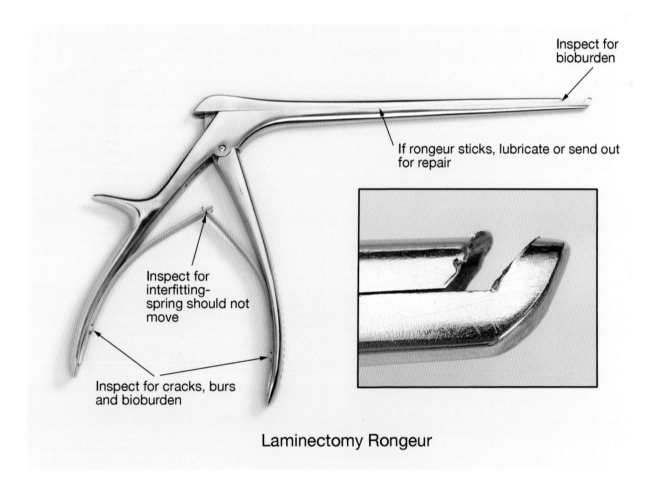

Inspect for bioburden

If rongeur sticks, lubricate or send out for repair

Inspect for interfitting-spring should not move

Inspect for cracks, burs and bioburden

Laminectomy Rongeur

Alexander-Farabeuf Periosteotome

Proper Name: Alexander-Farabeuf Periosteotome

Similar Instrument With Same Inspection: Matson

Length: 8.25" adult, 6" pediatric

Tip Definition:

- Double-ended with one end being a chisel shape, and the other being configured for scraping

Points of Inspection:

- Inspect both ends for cutting edge damage
- Handle should be smooth and clear

Criteria for Sharpness: Ability to scrape plastic dowel rod

Surgical Use: Scrape tissue and cartilage from ribs and bones

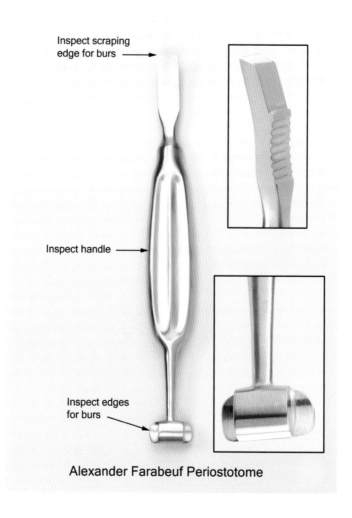

Inspect scraping edge for burs

Inspect handle

Inspect edges for burs

Alexander Farabeuf Periostotome

Finochietto Rib Spreader

Proper name: Finochietto Rib Spreader

Similar Instrument With Same Inspection: Harlen, Scapula, Buford

Length: 6", 8", 10", and 12" spread with straight arms

       8", 10", 12" spread with curved arms

Blade Definition: Various sizes, smooth and serrated blades

Points of inspections:

- Crank mechanism should be smooth
- Inspect for burs and surgical debris

Surgical Use: To spread open rib cage

Tray Assemble Tips: Due to weight of the instrument, the rib-spreader should be placed in the bottom of tray

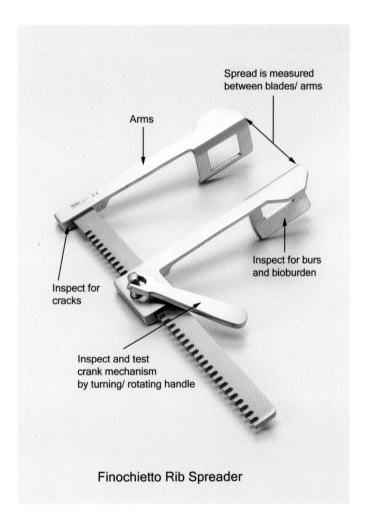

Finochietto Rib Spreader

Bailey Rib Contractor

Proper name: Bailey Rib Contractor

Similar Instruments: Bailey– Gibbon Rib Contractor-longer arms

Bailey Pediatric – small and lightweight

Tip Definition: 3 prongs on two arms

Tray Assemble Tips: Caution: <u>SHARPS RISK</u>.

Surgical use: To pull ribs back into place

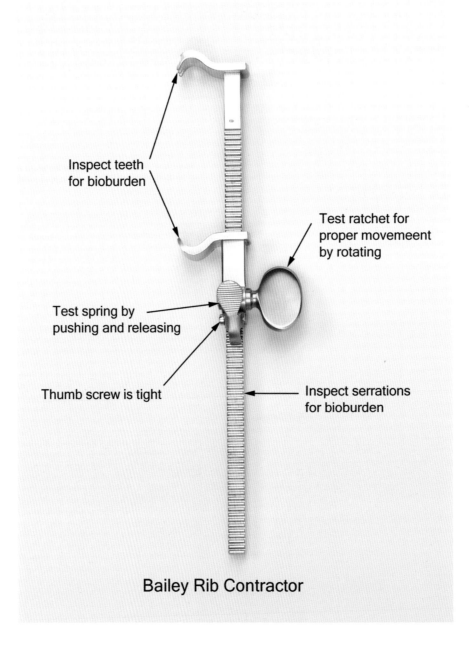

Inspect teeth
for bioburden

Test ratchet for
proper movemeent
by rotating

Test spring by
pushing and releasing

Thumb screw is tight

Inspect serrations
for bioburden

Bailey Rib Contractor

Lebsche Sternum Knife

Proper name: Lebsche Sternum Knife

Length: 10"

Criteria for sharpness: Plastic dowel rod

Tray Assemble Tips: Caution: <u>SHARPS RISK</u>.

Surgical use: To cut cartilage off the sternum

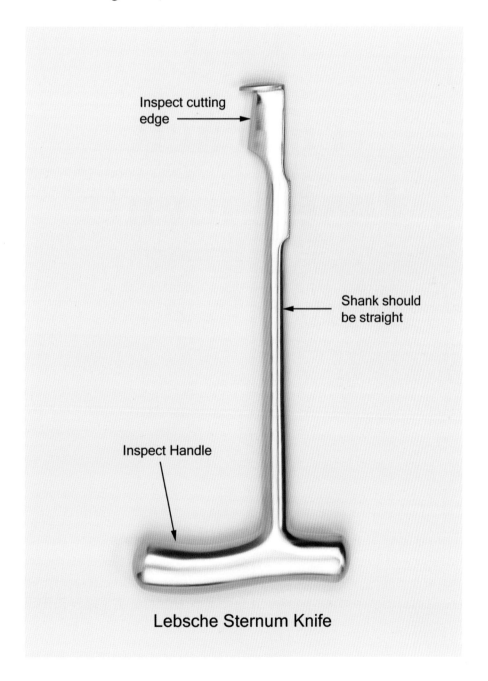

Lebsche Sternum Knife

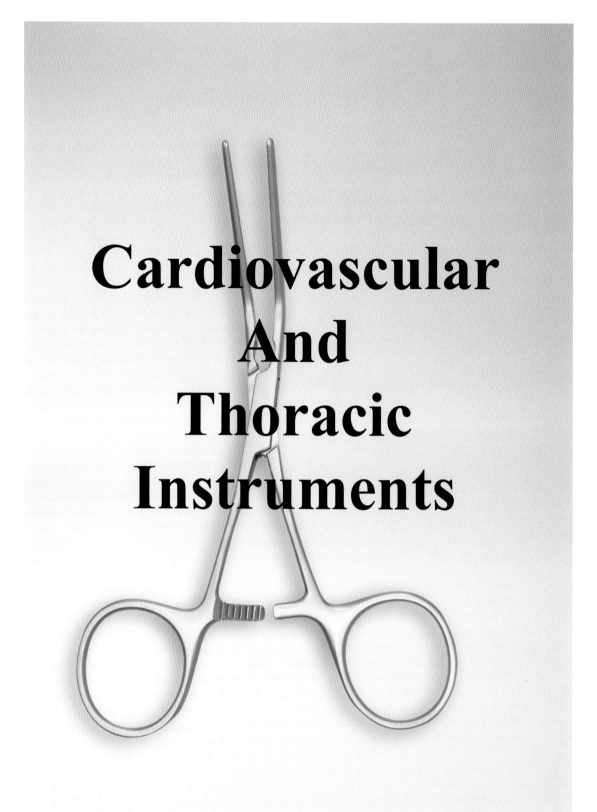

Cardiovascular And Thoracic Instruments

Cardiovascular Instruments/Thoracic Instruments – cardiovascular instruments are primarily used in surgical procedures relating to the heart and blood vessels, whereas thoracic instruments are used in surgical procedures relating to the organs located in the chest, especially the lungs.

Debakey Bulldog Clamp

Proper Name: Debakey Bulldog Clamp – Cross Action

Length: 7.5 cm, 8.5 cm, 10.5 cm, 12 cm

Tip/Jaw Definition: Straight and curved jaws (tips)

Tray Assemble Tips: Small clamps should be strung together with a stringer or kept in small cases

Surgical use: To occlude an artery while keeping vessels in tact

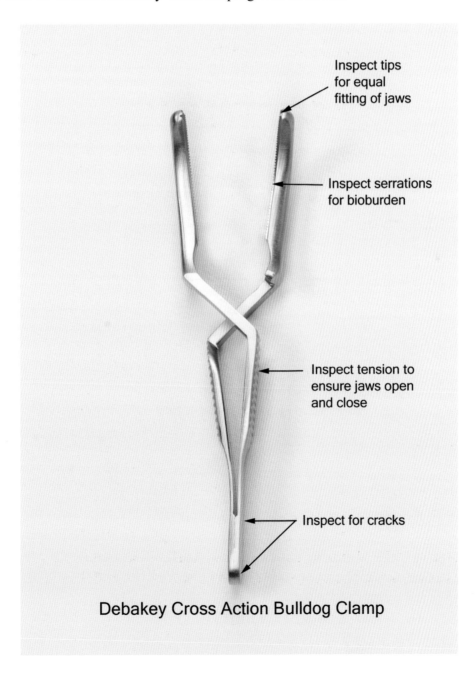

Inspect tips for equal fitting of jaws

Inspect serrations for bioburden

Inspect tension to ensure jaws open and close

Inspect for cracks

Debakey Cross Action Bulldog Clamp

Glover Bulldog Clamp

Proper Name: Glover Bulldog Clamp – With spring tension adjusting screw

Length: 7 cm, 8 cm, 9 cm, 11 cm

Tip Definition: Straight and curved jaws (tips)

Tray Assemble Tips: To prolong spring tension, it is recommended to loosen spring tension prior to sterilization

Surgical Use: To occlude and artery or vein, plus have control over tension

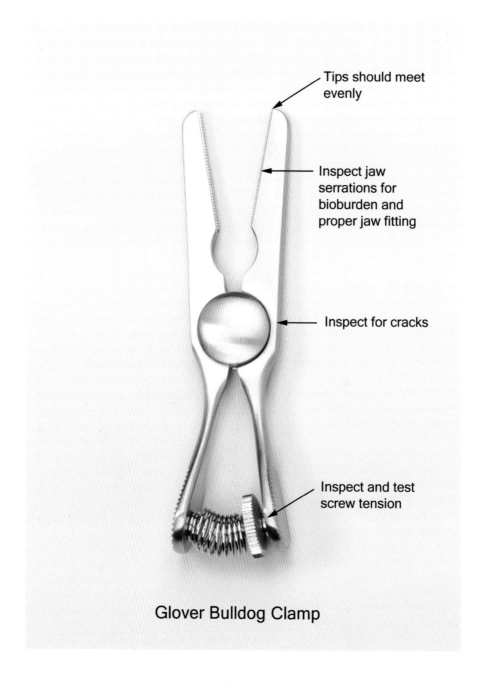

Tips should meet evenly

Inspect jaw serrations for bioburden and proper jaw fitting

Inspect for cracks

Inspect and test screw tension

Glover Bulldog Clamp

Debakey Ring Handled Bulldog Clamp

Proper Name: Debakey Ring Handled Bulldog Clamp

Length: Tip/Jaw definition: 5" Straight, 4.75" Curved, 4" 90°angle, 4.5" 45°angle, 4.75" S-Curved

Tray Assemble Tips: Sterilize with ratchet open

Surgical Use: To occlude vessels and arteries during vascular surgery

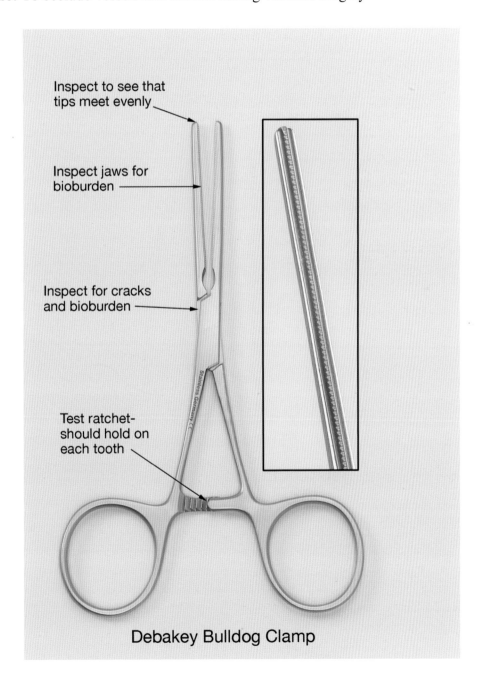

Inspect to see that tips meet evenly

Inspect jaws for bioburden

Inspect for cracks and bioburden

Test ratchet- should hold on each tooth

Debakey Bulldog Clamp

Debakey Vascular Clamp, Large

Proper Name: Debakey Vascular Clamp, Large

Length: 10", 10.5", 12.25", 12.75"

Tip/Jaw Definition: Slightly curved jaws

Tray Assemble Tips: Sterilize with ratchet open

Surgical Use: Vascular occlusion during aortic aneurism procedure

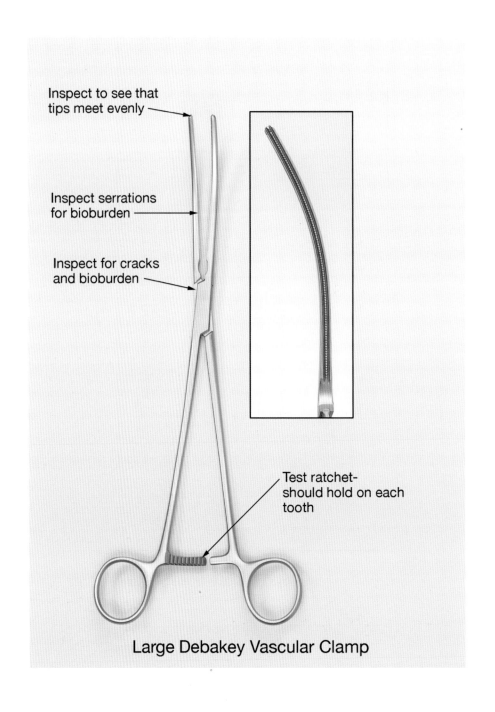

Inspect to see that tips meet evenly

Inspect serrations for bioburden

Inspect for cracks and bioburden

Test ratchet- should hold on each tooth

Large Debakey Vascular Clamp

Debakey Tangential Occlusion Clamp

Proper Name: Debakey Tangential Occlusion Clamp

Length: 8", 10", 10.25", 10.5", 11"

Tip/Jaw Definition: Atraumatic jaws

Tray Assemble Tips: Sterilize with jaws open

Surgical use: Vascular occlusion during cardiovascular surgery

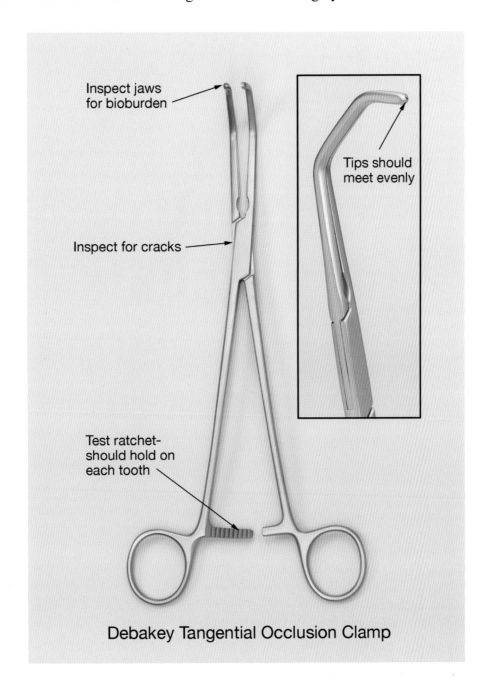

Inspect jaws for bioburden

Tips should meet evenly

Inspect for cracks

Test ratchet-should hold on each tooth

Debakey Tangential Occlusion Clamp

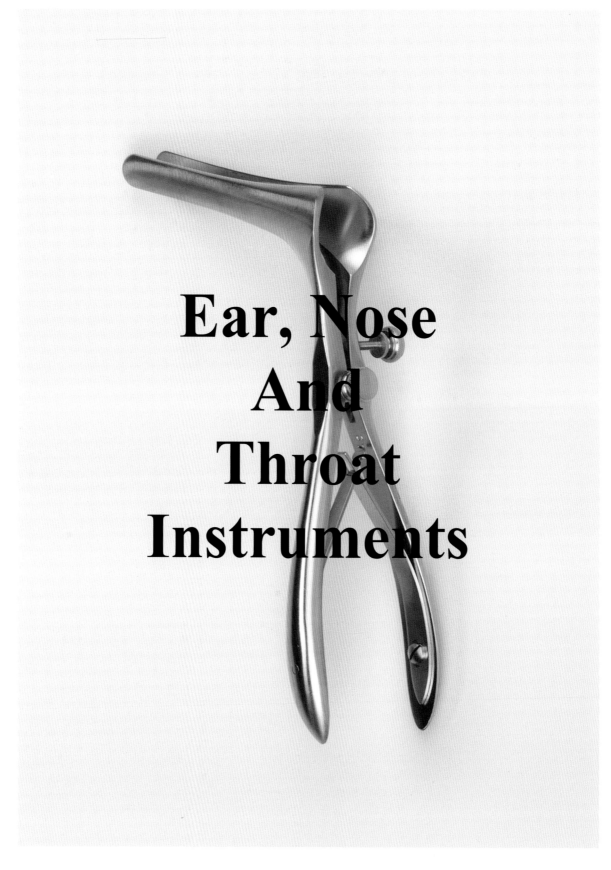

Ear, Nose
And
Throat
Instruments

ENT Instruments – used in surgical procedures related to the ear, nose, throat, and nearby parts of the head.

Jansen Ear Forcep

Proper Name: Jansen Ear Forcep

Similar Instruments with Same Inspections: Lucae and any other dressing forcep

Length: 5.5", 6.5"

Tip/Jaw Definition: Serrated tips and 1x2 teeth

Tray Assemble Tips: Sterilize with jaws open

Surgical Use: Manipulation of tissue and packing material for ENT procedures

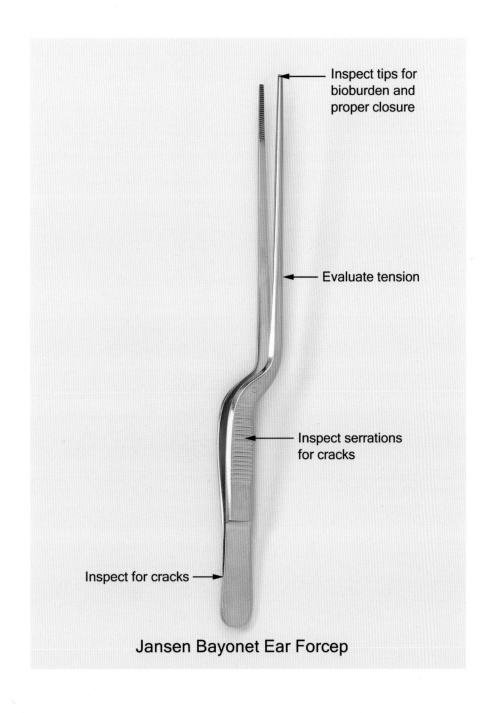

Inspect tips for bioburden and proper closure

Evaluate tension

Inspect serrations for cracks

Inspect for cracks

Jansen Bayonet Ear Forcep

Bowman Lacrimal Probe

Proper Name: Bowman Lacrimal Probe

Length: 5", Double ended, Sterling silver

Sizes: 0000-000, 00-0, 1-2, 3-4, 5-6, 7-8

Tray Assemble Tips: Due to instrument size it is recommended to keep it in a protective case

When very severe staining occurs, replacement is required

Surgical Use: Probing lacrimal duct

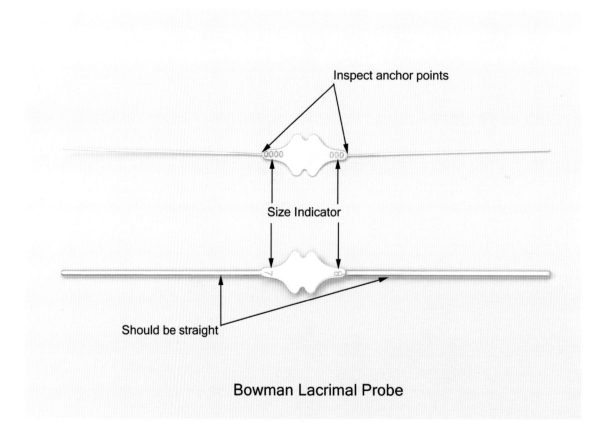

Bowman Lacrimal Probe

Fomon Retractor

Proper Name: Fomon Retractor

Similar Instruments with Same Inspections: Cottle Retractor

Length: 6.5"

Tip Definition: Two prongs 11mm wide with 2 ball prongs

Tray Assemble Tips:

- Prongs can penetrate bottom of mesh trays and become damaged

- Protective case or pouch is recommended

Surgical Use: Retraction during ENT procedures

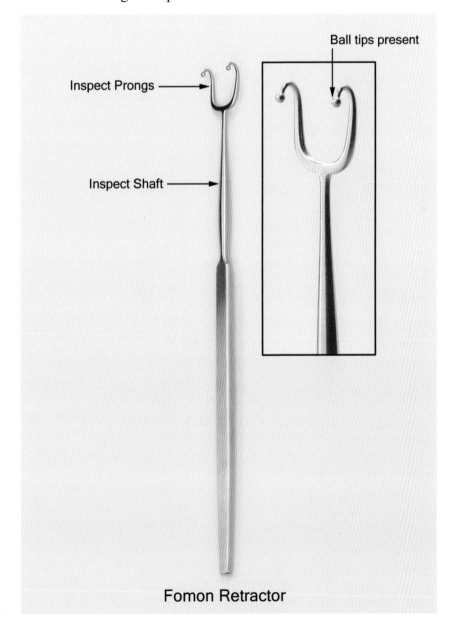

Ball tips present

Inspect Prongs

Inspect Shaft

Fomon Retractor

Aufricht Retractor

Proper Name: Aufricht Retractor

Length: 6.5" solid blades, 6.5" fenestrated blades

Tip Definition: Single blade

Tray Assemble Tips:

- Protective case or pouch is recommended

Surgical Use: Retraction during nasal procedures

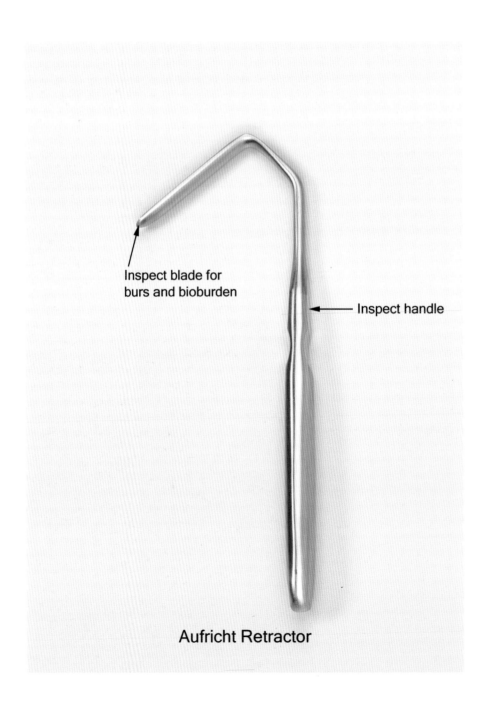

Inspect blade for burs and bioburden

Inspect handle

Aufricht Retractor

Joseph Hook

Proper Name: Joseph Hook

Length: 6.25"

Tip definition: Single hook, double hook 2mm, 5mm, 7mm, 10mm. Measured between hooks

Tray Assemble Tips: Caution: <u>SHARPS RISK.</u> Use tip protectors

- Dual prong retractors and skin hooks possess a sharps risk
- Prongs can penetrate bottom of mesh trays and become damaged

Surgical use: Retraction of soft tissue

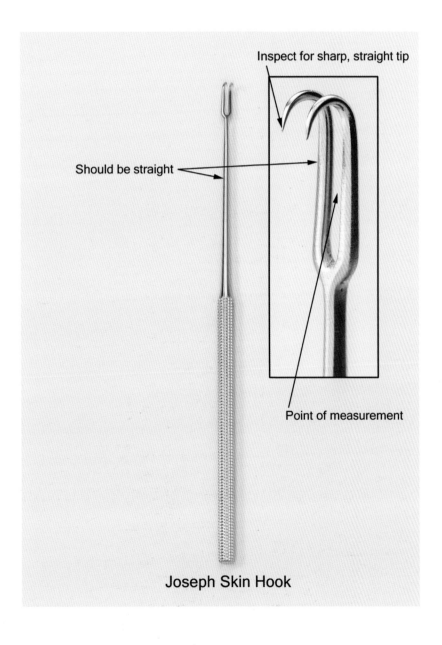

Joseph Skin Hook

Hartman Ear Specula

Proper Name: Hartman Ear Specula, Set of 3

Similar Instruments:

- Gruber
- Toynbee (set of 3)
- Farrior (set of 9)

Diameter: 3mm, 4mm, 5mm

Tip Definition: Round, Oval, Angled

Surgical Use: For examination of the ear

Tray Assemble Tips: Ear specula come in sets

Always verify the sizes

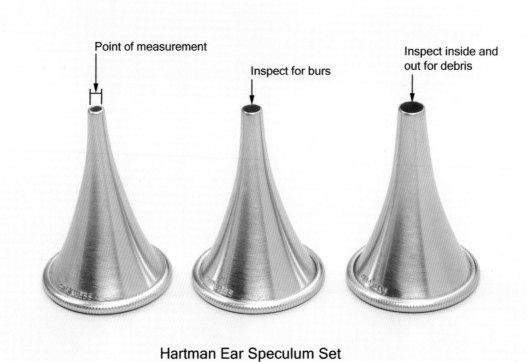

Hartman Ear Speculum Set

Hartman Ear Forcep

Proper Name: Hartman Ear Forcep

Similar Instruments with Same Inspection:

- Littauer ear Forcep
- Hartman Alligator Forcep
- Hartmann Royes Forcep
- Hoffmann Ear Forcep

Length: 5"

Tip/Jaw Definition: Delicate serrated jaws, 2.4mm x 6mm

Tray Assemble Tips: Sterilize with jaws open

Surgical Use: To grasp or manipulate tissue during nasal or ear procedures

Also used for removal of foreign bodies

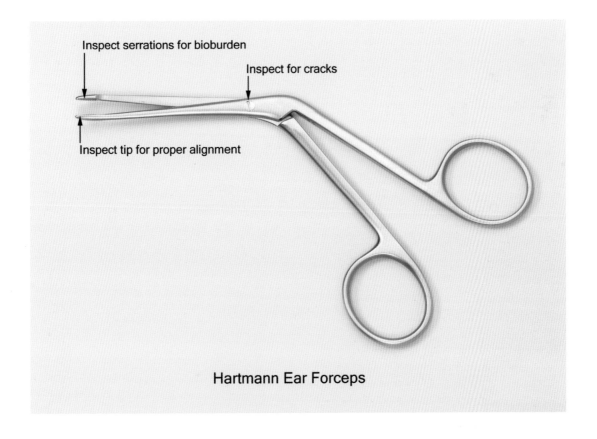

Inspect serrations for bioburden

Inspect for cracks

Inspect tip for proper alignment

Hartmann Ear Forceps

Hartman Alligator Forcep

Proper Name: Hartman Alligator Forcep

Length: Shaft lengths; 3", 4", 5", 7"

Tip/Jaw Definition: Serrated jaws

Tray Assemble Tips: Inspect jaw hinge with magnification looking for micro cracks

Surgical Use: Use for grasping tissue during ENT procedures

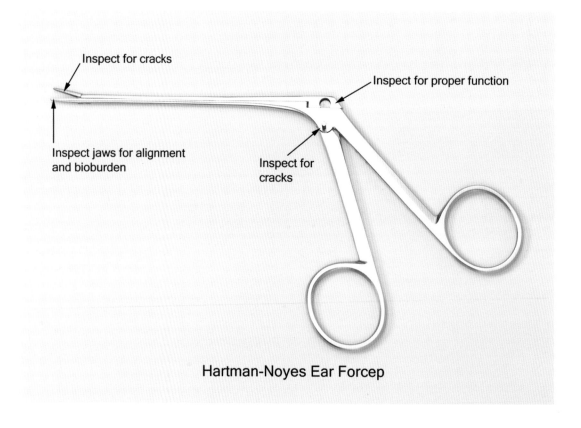

Hartman-Noyes Ear Forcep

Killian Septum Speculum

Proper Name: Killian Septum Speculum

Similar Instruments with same Inspections: Cottle Speculum, Vienna Speculum

Length: 6"

Tip/Jaw Definition: Blades of 2", 2.5", 3", 3.5"

Surgical Use: For nasal retraction and examination

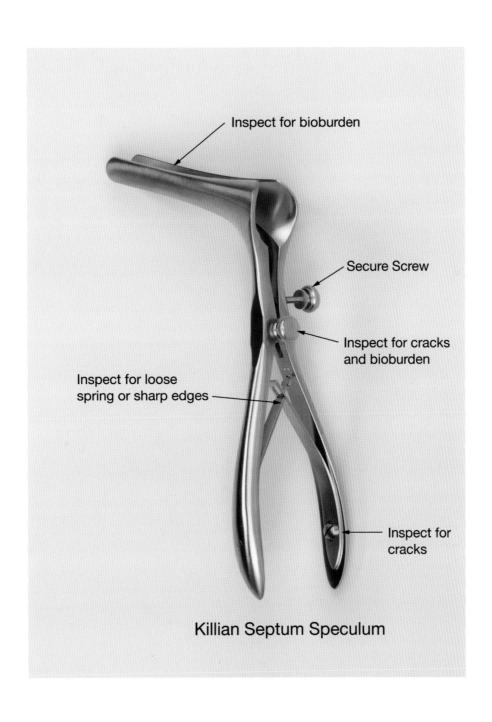

Inspect for bioburden

Secure Screw

Inspect for cracks and bioburden

Inspect for loose spring or sharp edges

Inspect for cracks

Killian Septum Speculum

Bruening Snare

Proper Name: Bruening Snare

Other Common Patterns:

- Krause Nasal Snare
- Bruening Ear Snare
- Eve Tonsil Snare
- Beck Schenk Tonsil Snare
- Tyding Tonsil Snare

Length: 9"

Tip Definition: Small, fine tube with snare wire that moves in and out

Tray Assemble Tips: Be sure wire is properly secured and always provide additional wires

Surgical use: To remove tonsils

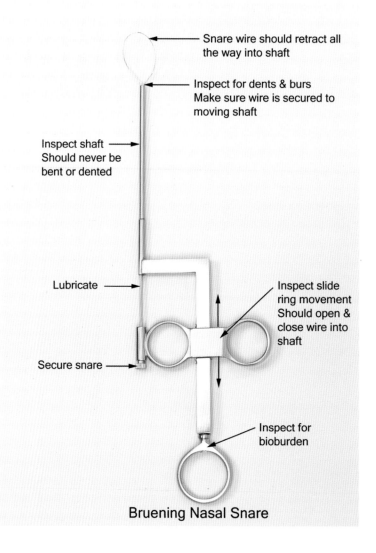

Bruening Nasal Snare

Ballenger Swivel Knife

Proper Name: Ballenger Swivel Knife

Similar Instruments with same Inspections: None

Length: 7.75"

Tip Definition: Movable/swinging, cutting edge in various widths: 3mm, 4mm, 5mm

Straight shaft or bayonet shaft

Criteria for Sharpness: Knife edge should cut into plastic dowel rod

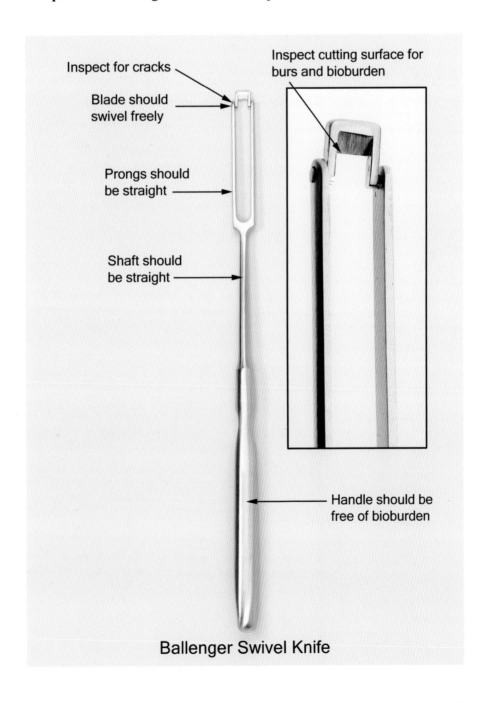

Inspect for cracks

Blade should swivel freely

Prongs should be straight

Shaft should be straight

Inspect cutting surface for burs and bioburden

Handle should be free of bioburden

Ballenger Swivel Knife

Jansen-Middleton Septum Forcep

Proper Name: Jansen-Middleton Septum Forcep

Similar Instruments with same Inspections: None

Length: 7.5"

Tip Definition: Two types of Jaws:

- Spoon/cup shaped
- Through punch cutting

Criteria for Sharpness: Jaws should imprint evenly into index card

Surgical Use: To cut/grasp septum

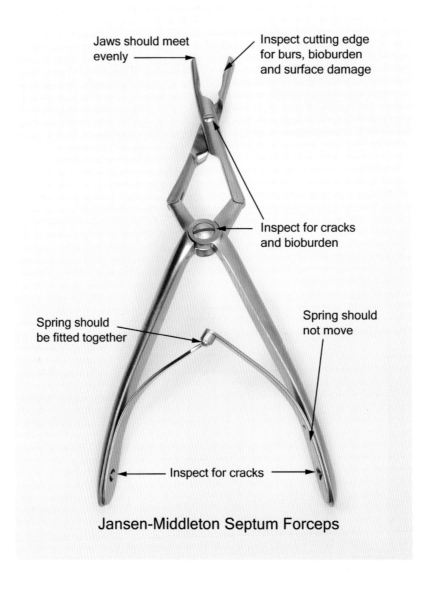

Jansen-Middleton Septum Forceps

Caplan Nasal Bone Scissor

Proper Name: Caplan Nasal Bone Scissor

Other Names: Angled Nasal Scissor

Similar Instruments With Same Inspection: McIndoe Bone Cutting Forcep, Kazanjian Nasal Cutting Forcep

Blade Definition: Serrated blades with double-action and angled design

Length: 8"

Surgical Use: Cutting of nasal bone and cartilage

Sharpness Test Standard: Red scissor test material

Tray Assembly Tips: Keep rings slightly separated and tips of scissors going in same direction

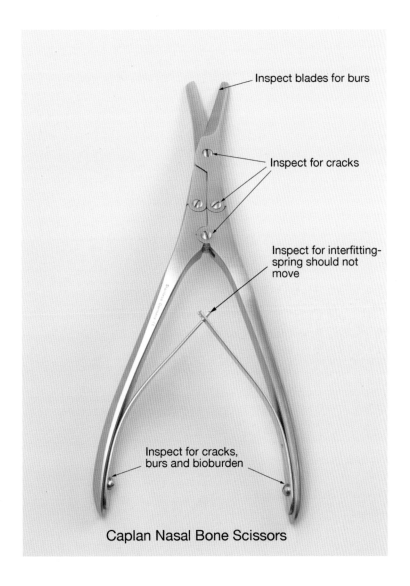

Caplan Nasal Bone Scissors

Cottle Dorsal Scissor

Proper Name: Cottle Dorsal Scissor

Other Names: Angled Scissor, Angled Mayo

Similar Instruments With Same Inspection: Fomon Scissor

Blade Definition: Round blades

Length: 5.5" and 6.5"

Surgical Use: Nasal dissection procedures

Sharpness Test Standard: Red scissor test material

Tray Assembly Tips: Keep rings slightly separated and tips of scissors going in same direction

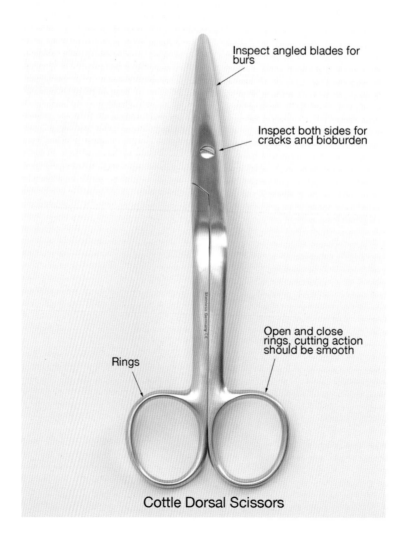

Inspect angled blades for burs

Inspect both sides for cracks and bioburden

Open and close rings, cutting action should be smooth

Rings

Cottle Dorsal Scissors

Barnhill Adenoid Curette

Proper Name: Barnhill Adenoid Curette

Similar Instruments with same Inspections: Vogel Curette

Length: 8.5"

Tip Definition: Cutting blade widths: 11mm, 13mm, 15mm, 17mm, 19mm

7mm blade is infant size and is known as a Vogel Curette

Criteria for Sharpness: Inside of blade should cut into plastic dowel rod

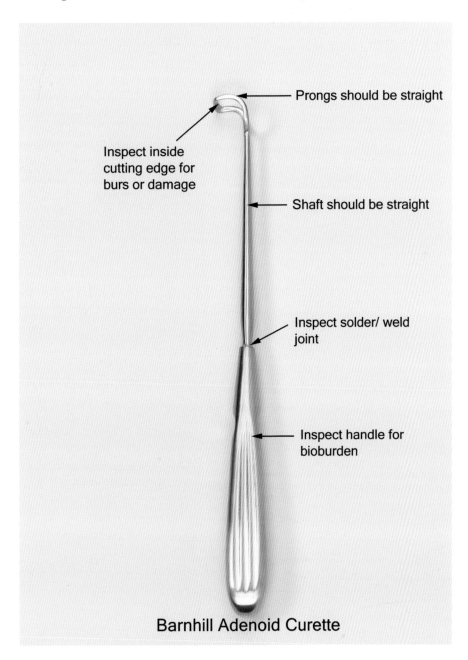

Prongs should be straight

Inspect inside cutting edge for burs or damage

Shaft should be straight

Inspect solder/ weld joint

Inspect handle for bioburden

Barnhill Adenoid Curette

Fomon Periosteal Elevator

Proper Name: Fomon Periosteal Elevator

Similar Instruments with same Inspections: Freer, Cottle Mckenty, Joseph Selden

Length: 6.25"

Tip Definition: Blade is slightly curved and single-ended

Freer elevator is double-ended, with one blade sharp and one blade blunt

Points of Inspection: Inspect instrument for bioburden

Criteria for Sharpness: Should be able to scrape plastic dowel rod

Surgical Use: Used to separate the periosteum

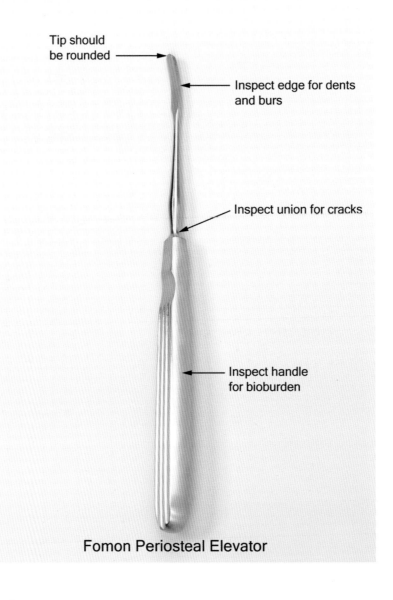

Tip should be rounded

Inspect edge for dents and burs

Inspect union for cracks

Inspect handle for bioburden

Fomon Periosteal Elevator

OB/GYN
Instruments

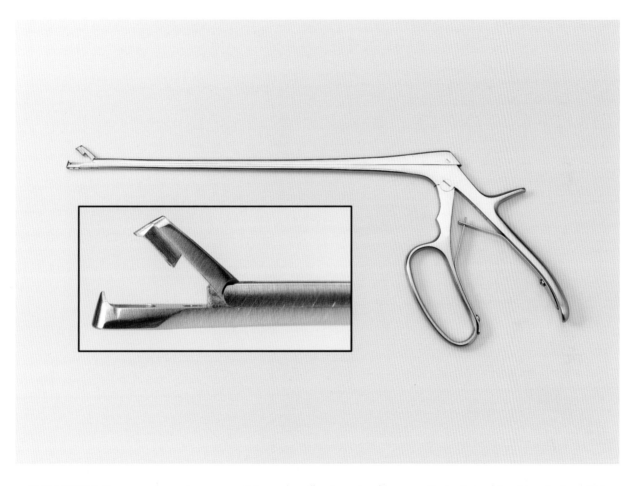

OB/GYN Instruments – used in surgical practices related to the basic health of the female reproductive system and childbirth.

Gutmann Vaginal Speculum

Proper Name: Gutmann Vaginal Speculum

Length: Blade size, 1.375" x 4"

Surgical Use: To retract vaginal walls

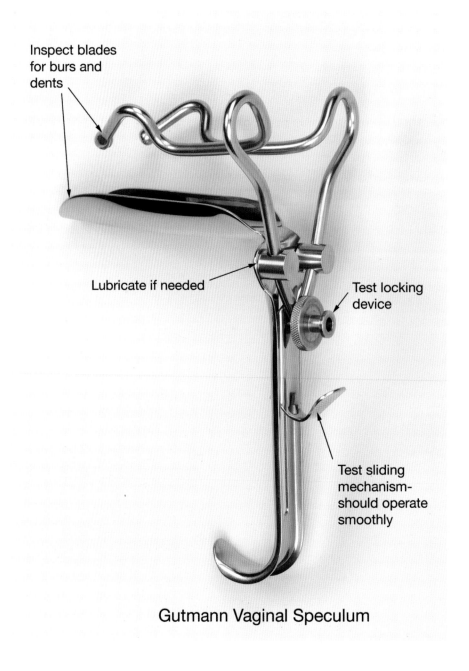

Inspect blades for burs and dents

Lubricate if needed

Test locking device

Test sliding mechanism- should operate smoothly

Gutmann Vaginal Speculum

Auvard Weighted Speculum

Proper Name: Auvard Weighted Speculum

Similar Names: Steiner-Auvard

Weights: 2lbs, 2.5lbs, 3lbs

Tip Definition: None

Blades:

- 1.5" W x 3.25" L, 75º angle

- 1.375" W x 4" L, tapered at a 45º angle

- 1.25" W x 5.25" L, slightly curved up at a 90º angle

Tray Assemble Tips: If instrument is made of chrome, process separately or replace with stainless version

Always put speculum on bottom of tray due to weight of instrument

Surgical Use: Posterior vaginal wall retraction

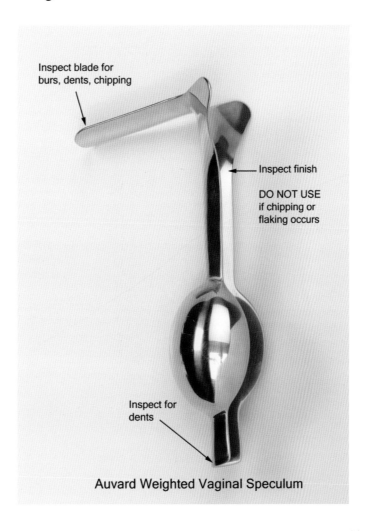

Auvard Weighted Vaginal Speculum

Jackson Vaginal Retractor

Proper Name: Jackson Vaginal Retractor

Similar Instruments with same Inspections: Eastman Retractor, Doyen Retractor

Length: 7"

Tip/Blade Definition:

- 1.5" W x 3" L
- 1.5" W x 3.5" L
- 1.5" W x 4" L

Surgical Use: Retraction of vaginal walls

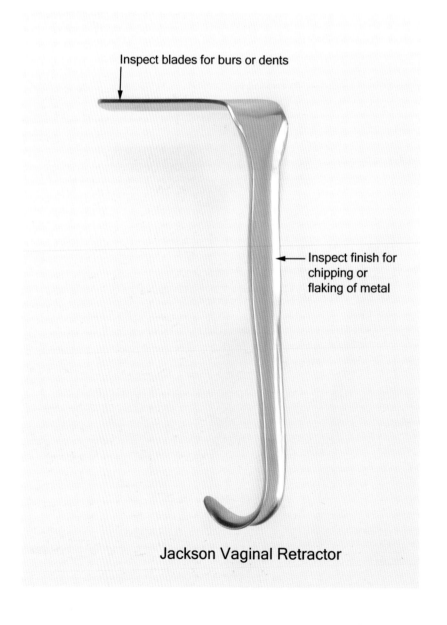

Inspect blades for burs or dents

Inspect finish for chipping or flaking of metal

Jackson Vaginal Retractor

Delee Universal Bladder Retractor

Proper Name: Delee Universal Bladder Retractor

Length: 9.5"

Blade Dimension: 2" deep x 2.75" wide, also available in left and right design

Surgical Use: Retraction of bladder during C-section

Tray Assemble Tips: Caution: If instrument is made of chrome, process separately or replace with stainless version

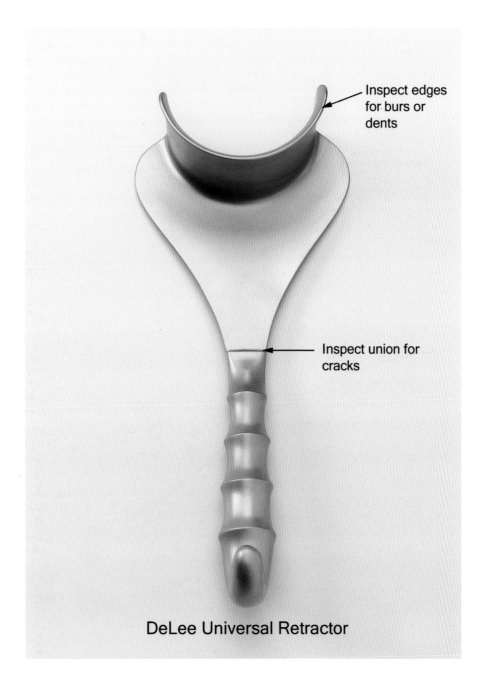

DeLee Universal Retractor

Hank Uterine Dilators

Proper Name: Hank Uterine Dilators

Similar Instruments: Hegar, Pratt

Length: 11" various diameters

Tip Definition: Each end of a dilator is a different diameter. The diameter is noted in French scale, which is numerically marked on each dilator end

Surgical Use: To dilate the cervix

Tray Assemble Tips: Usually assembled in a set of six

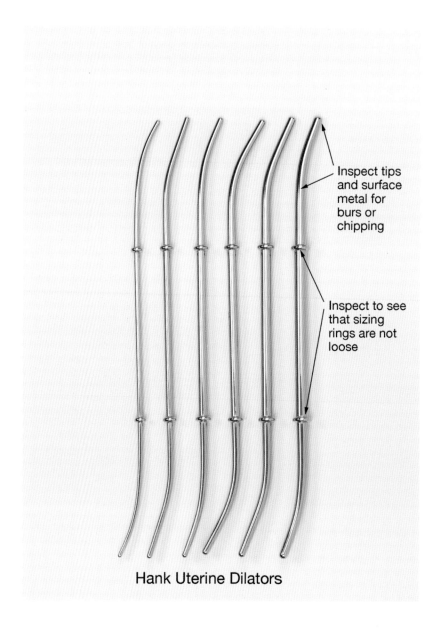

Inspect tips and surface metal for burs or chipping

Inspect to see that sizing rings are not loose

Hank Uterine Dilators

Goodell Uterine Dilator

Proper Name: Goodell Uterine Dilator

Length: 11" or 13"

Tip/Blade Definition: Distal tips have very large serrations

Surgical Use: Dilates the cervix

Tray Assemble Tips: Caution: If Goodell Dilator is made of chrome, process separately or replace with stainless version

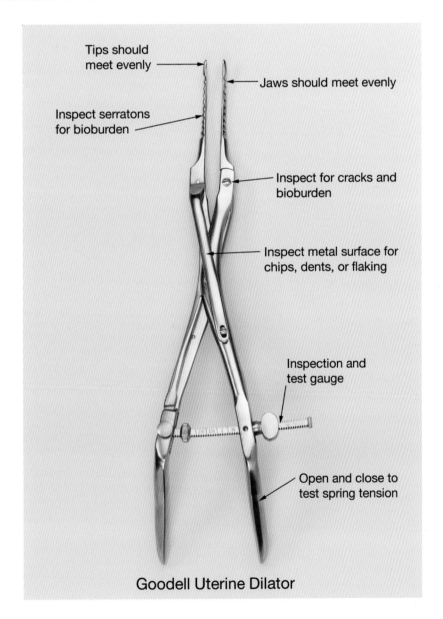

Goodell Uterine Dilator

Bill Traction Handle

Proper Name: Bill Traction Handle

Length: 4.5"

Surgical use: Attaches to obstetrical forcep for application of traction during delivery

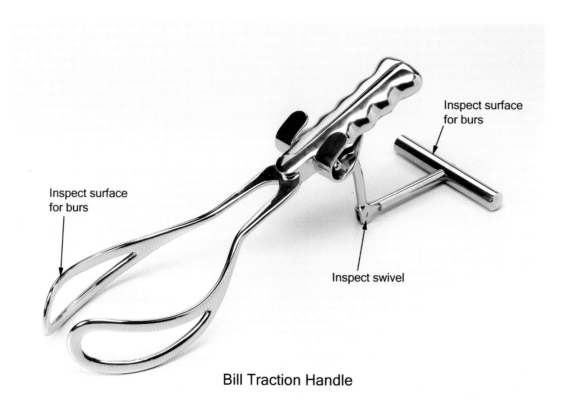

Inspect surface for burs

Inspect surface for burs

Inspect swivel

Bill Traction Handle

Iowa Trumpet Pudendal Needle Guide

Proper Name: Iowa Trumpet Pudendal Needle Guide

Length: 5.5"

Surgical Use: Insert needle into Trumpet end; allows for needle extension while distal tip protects against puncture from sharp needle

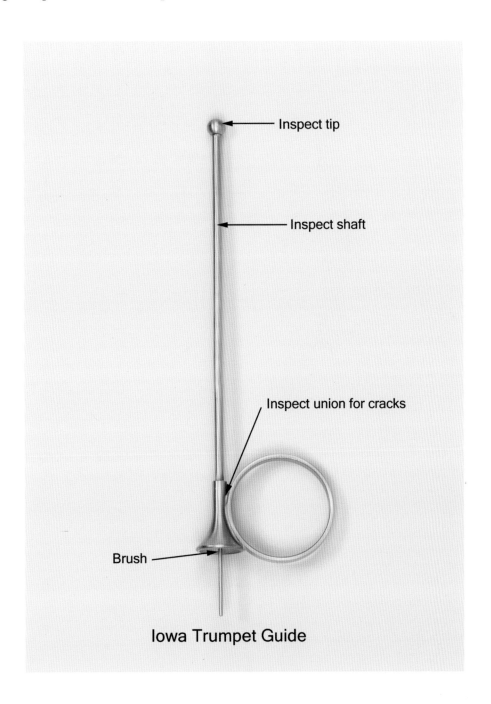

Iowa Trumpet Guide

Simpson Obstetrical Forcep

Proper Name: Simpson Obstetrical Forcep

Similar Instruments: DeLee, Elliott, Piper, Kielland, Luikart, Mclean

Length: 12" or 14"

Tip Definition: Open fenestrated blades

Tray Assemble Tips: place in bottom of tray due to weight of forceps

Surgical Use: Blades are used to extract newborn during vaginal delivery

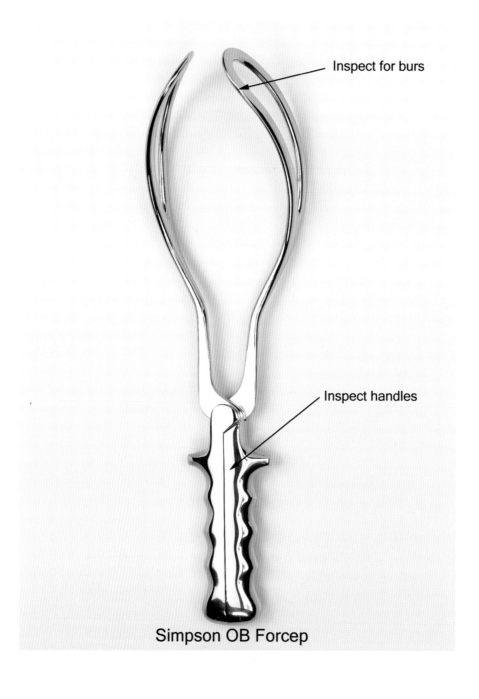

Inspect for burs

Inspect handles

Simpson OB Forcep

Braun Episiotomy Scissor

Proper Name: Braun Episiotomy Scissor

Similar Instruments: None

Length: 5.5" and 8.5"

Tip Definition: Very blunted scissor blades

Surgical Use: Used in vaginal deliveries

Tray Assemble Tips: Sterilize with rings open

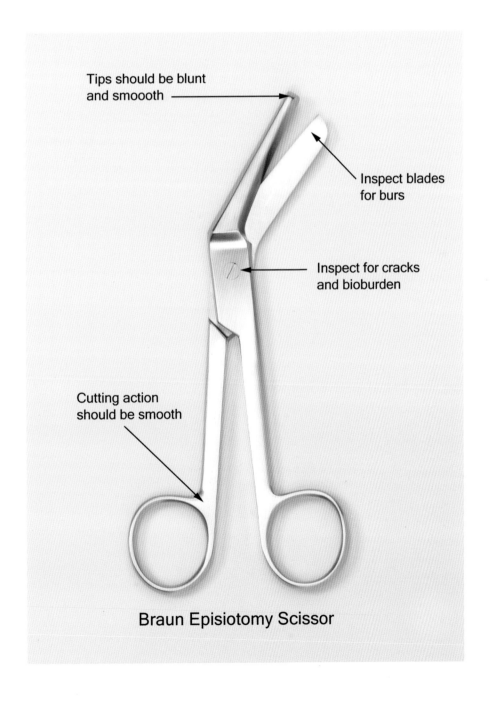

Braun Episiotomy Scissor

Sims Uterine Scissor

Proper Name: Sims Uterine Scissor

Other Names: Uterine Scissor

Similar Instruments With Same Inspection: Kelly Uterine Scissor, Mayo Uterine Scissor

Blade Definition: Two scissor blades with sharp/sharp points, sharp/blunt points, or blunt/blunt points

Length: 8"

Surgical Use: To cut the uterus

Sharpness Test Standard: Red test material

Tray Assembly Tips: Keep rings slightly separated and tips of scissors going in same direction

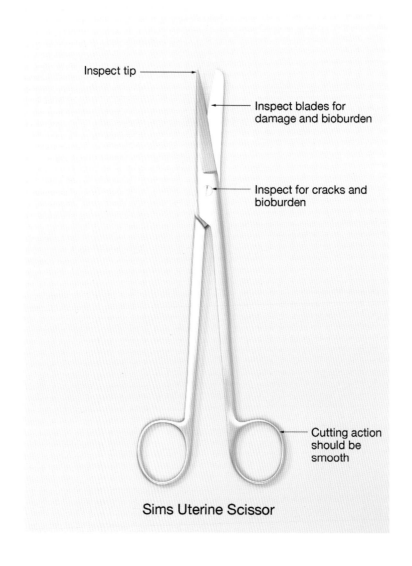

Sims Uterine Scissor

Novak Uterine Curette

Proper Name: Novak Uterine Curette

Similar Instruments: None

Length: 9.75", 4mm or 2mm diameter

Tip Definition: Slightly curved cannulated tip with serrated edges surrounding the opening

Surgical Use: Used to obtain uterine biopsy samples

Tray Assemble Tips: Always put stylet in tray with curette

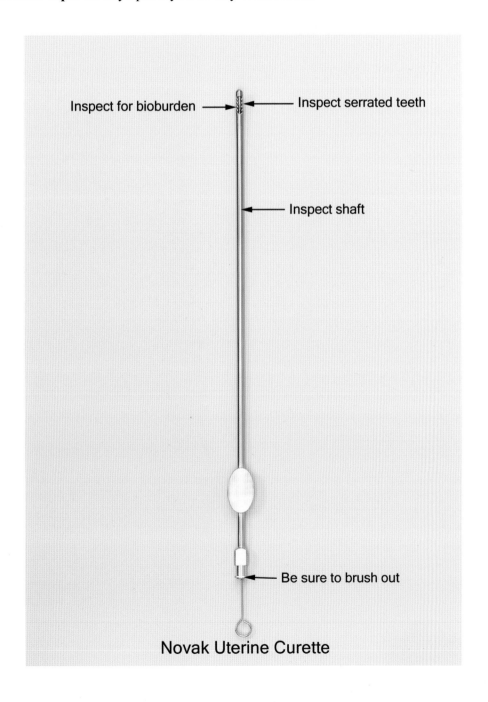

Inspect for bioburden — Inspect serrated teeth

— Inspect shaft

— Be sure to brush out

Novak Uterine Curette

Kevorkian Younge Endocervical Biopsy Forcep

Proper Name: Kevorkian Younge Endocervical Biopsy Forcep

Similar Instruments: None

Length: 12"

Tip Definition: Semi-sharp rectangular tip with basket

Surgical Use: To obtain a sample of the cervix

Tray Assemble Tips: Sterilize with jaw open

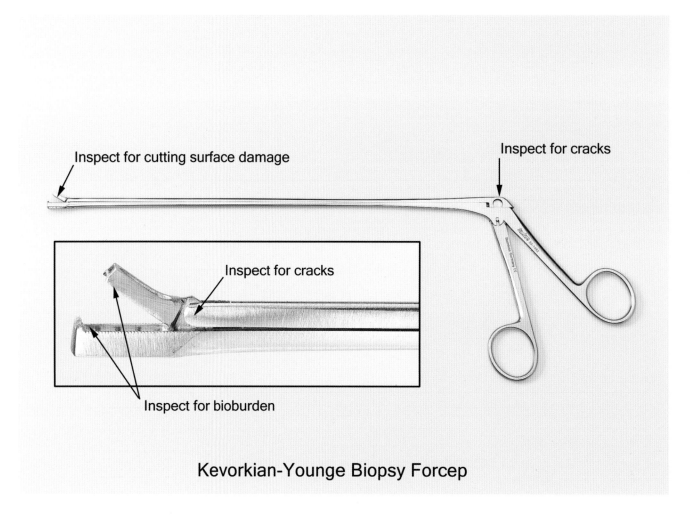

Kevorkian-Younge Biopsy Forcep

Kogan Endocervical Speculum

Proper Name: Kogan Endocervical Speculum

Similar Instruments: None

Length: 9.5"

Tip Definition: Two loop fenestrated jaws with outside serrations

Surgical Use: Endocervical retraction

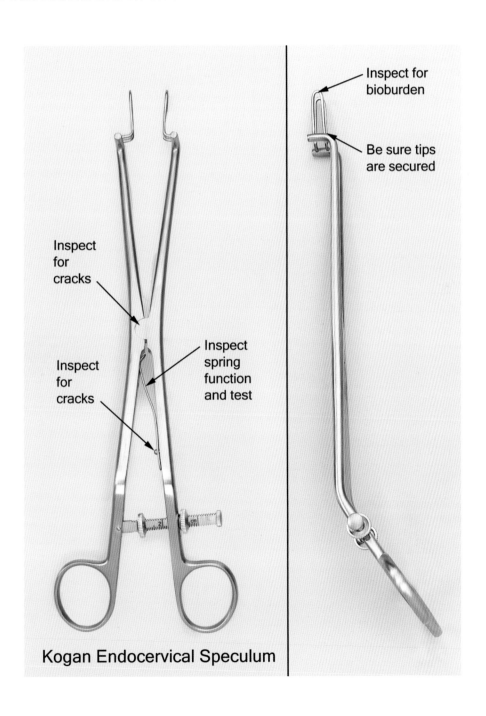

Inspect for bioburden

Be sure tips are secured

Inspect for cracks

Inspect for cracks

Inspect spring function and test

Kogan Endocervical Speculum

Heaney Hysterectomy Forcep

Proper Name: Heaney Hysterectomy Forcep

Other Names: Ballentine, double tooth

Similar Instruments With Same Inspection: Heaney-Ballentine, Garland Forcep

Jaw Definition: Serrated jaw with one or two notched teeth

Length: 8.25" and 9.75"

Surgical Use: Clamping onto the uterus

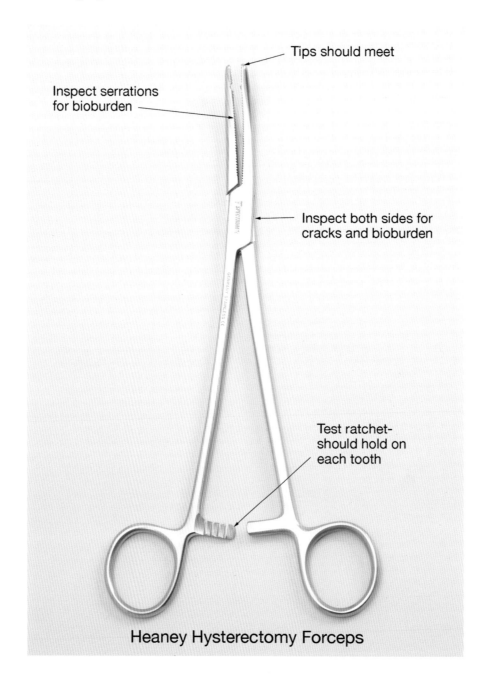

Tips should meet

Inspect serrations for bioburden

Inspect both sides for cracks and bioburden

Test ratchet- should hold on each tooth

Heaney Hysterectomy Forceps

Jacobs Uterine Vulsellum Forcep

Proper Name: Jacobs Uterine Vulsellum Forcep

Similar Instruments: Teale, Kelly, Schroeder, Skene, Vulsellum Forceps

Length: 8.5"

Tip Definition: 2x2 teeth with serrations below teeth

Surgical Use: Grasping and manipulating of the uterus

Tray Assemble Tips: Sterilize with ratchet open

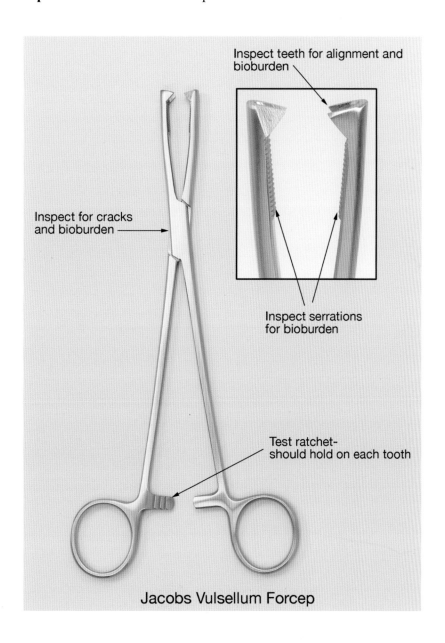

Inspect teeth for alignment and bioburden

Inspect for cracks and bioburden

Inspect serrations for bioburden

Test ratchet- should hold on each tooth

Jacobs Vulsellum Forcep

Schroeder Uterine Tenaculum

Proper Name: Schroeder Uterine Tenaculum

Similar Instruments: Kahn, Duplay, Adair, Staude, Barrett, Jarcho, Skene

Length: 9.5"

Tip Definition: Two sharp prongs

Surgical Use: Grasping and manipulating of the cervix

Tray Assemble Tips: Caution: SHARPS RISK. Distal tips contain two sharp points

Sterilize with ratchet open

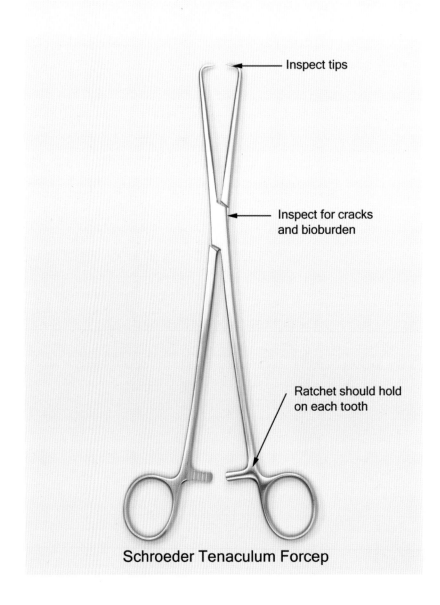

Inspect tips

Inspect for cracks and bioburden

Ratchet should hold on each tooth

Schroeder Tenaculum Forcep

Tischler Biopsy Forcep

Proper Name: Tischler Biopsy Forcep

Similar Instruments: Shubert, Thoms-Gaylor, Burke, Townsend, Eppendorfer, Wittner

Length: 9"

Criteria for Sharpness: One thickness of a facial tissue should punch clean

Surgical Use: To obtain biopsy sample of the cervix

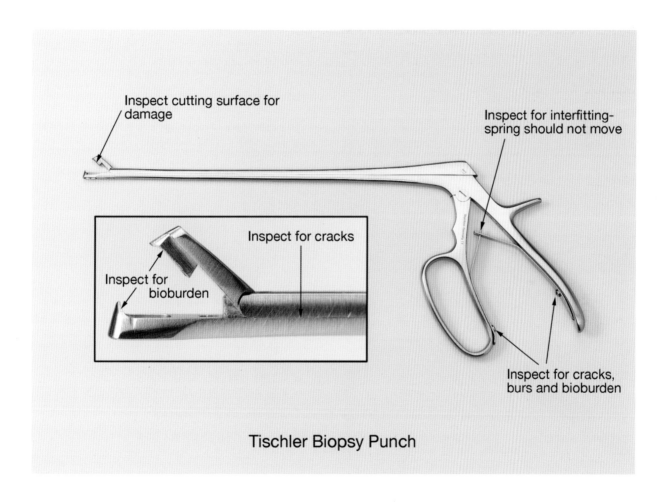

Inspect cutting surface for damage

Inspect for interfitting-spring should not move

Inspect for cracks

Inspect for bioburden

Inspect for cracks, burs and bioburden

Tischler Biopsy Punch

Kevorkian-Younge Biopsy Curette

Proper Name: Kevorkian-Younge Biopsy Curette

Similar Instruments: Heany, Sims

Type: Curette with basket and without basket

Length: 12"

Criteria for Sharpness: Plastic dowel rod should scrape

Surgical Use: To obtain a biopsy of the cervix

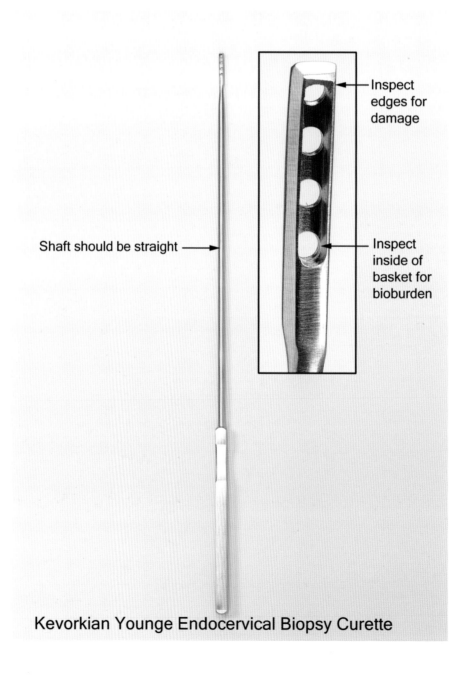

Shaft should be straight →

Inspect edges for damage

Inspect inside of basket for bioburden

Kevorkian Younge Endocervical Biopsy Curette

Circumcision Clamps

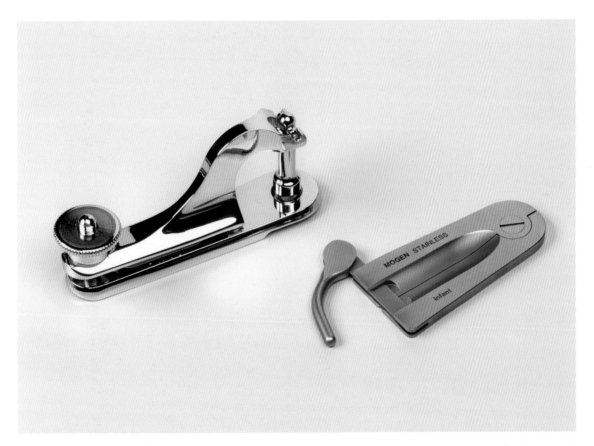

Circumcision Clamps – used to surgically remove the foreskin of the penis.

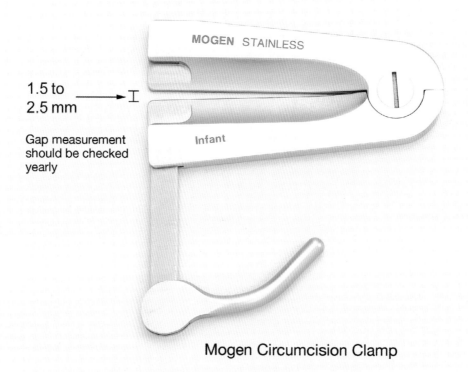

1.5 to
2.5 mm

Gap measurement
should be checked
yearly

Mogen Circumcision Clamp

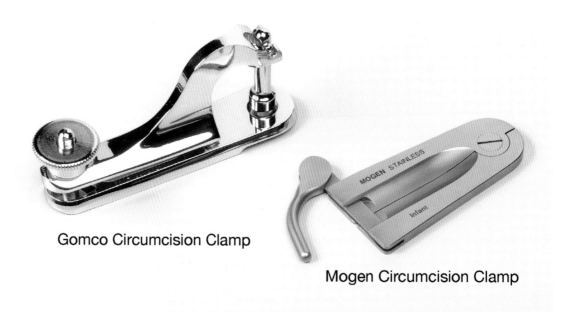

Gomco Circumcision Clamp

Mogen Circumcision Clamp

236

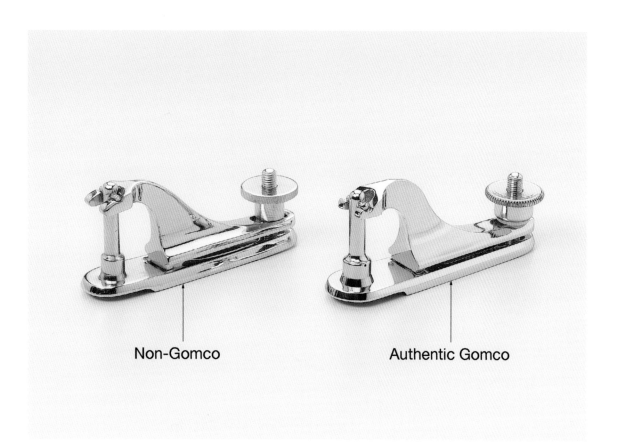

Non-Gomco   Authentic Gomco

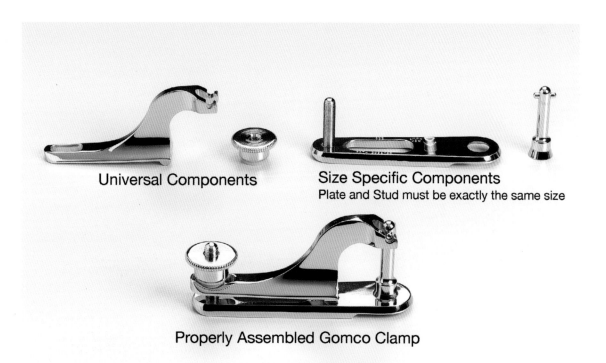

Universal Components   Size Specific Components
                             Plate and Stud must be exactly the same size

Properly Assembled Gomco Clamp

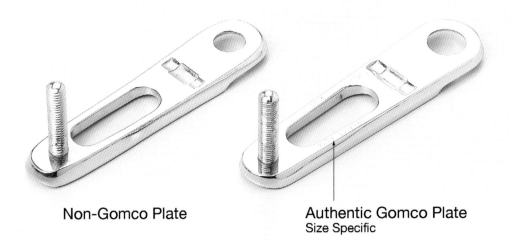

Non-Gomco Plate

Authentic Gomco Plate
Size Specific

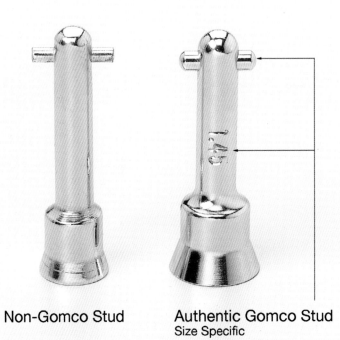

Non-Gomco Stud

Authentic Gomco Stud
Size Specific

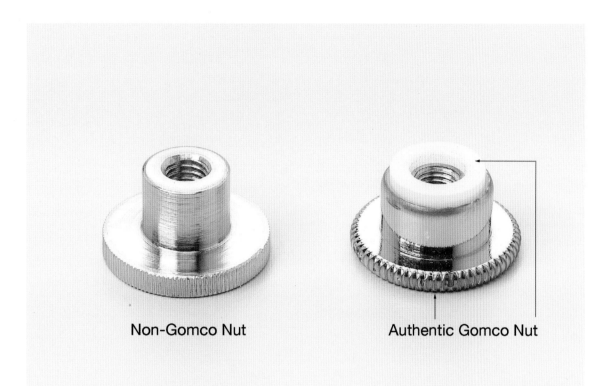

Non-Gomco Nut   Authentic Gomco Nut

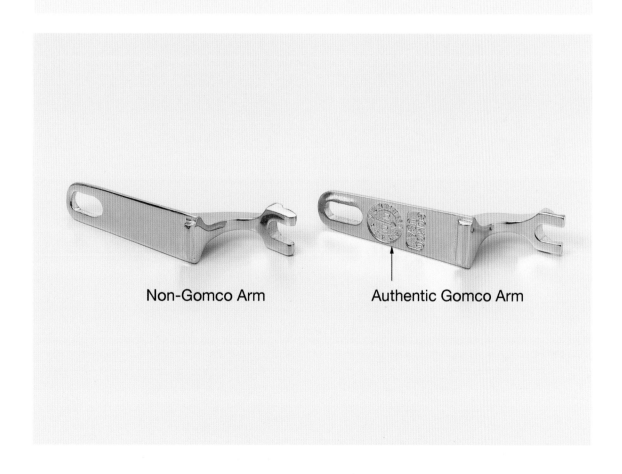

Non-Gomco Arm   Authentic Gomco Arm

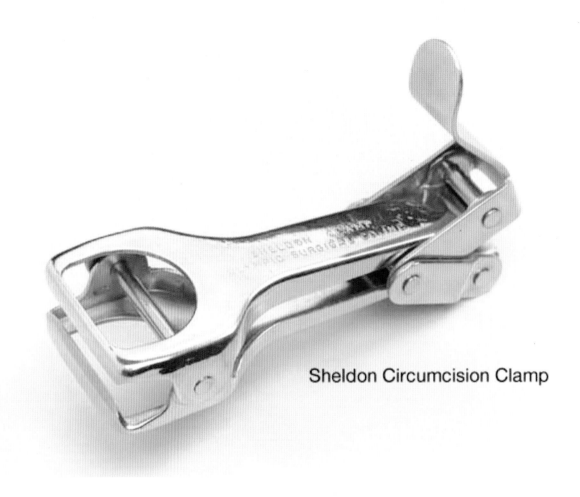

Sheldon Circumcision Clamp

The Sheldon Circumcision Clamp is a rarely used instrument. It is no longer being produced however; some practitioners still use the device.

Ophthalmic Instruments

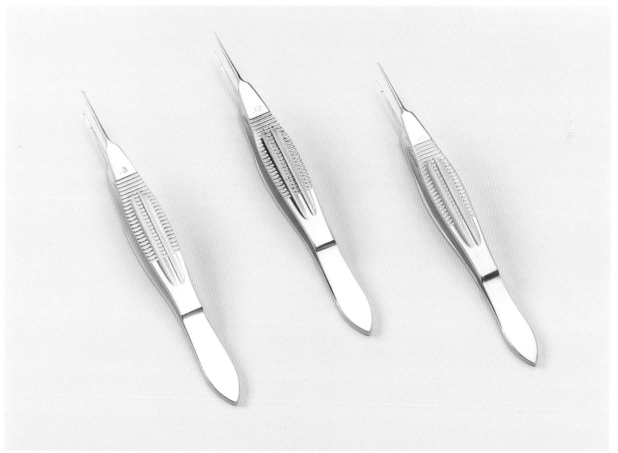

Ophthalmic Instruments – used in treating disorders and diseases of the eye.

Desmarres Chalazion Retractor

Proper Name: Desmarres Chalazion Retractor

Length: 5.5"

Tip/Blade Definition: Blade sizes – 11mm, 13mm, 15mm, 18mm

Surgical Use: Eye lid retraction/dissection

Tray Assemble Tips: *DELICATE INSTRUMENT*; should be placed in a protective sterilization case with silicon mat

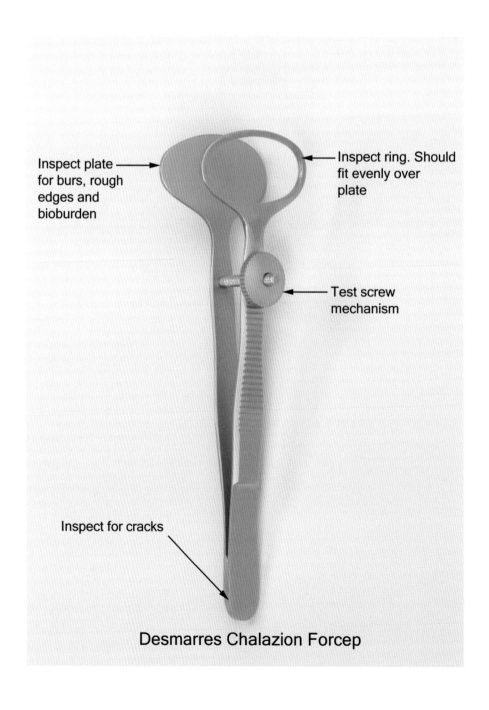

Inspect plate for burs, rough edges and bioburden

Inspect ring. Should fit evenly over plate

Test screw mechanism

Inspect for cracks

Desmarres Chalazion Forcep

Iris Scissor

Proper Name: Iris Scissor

Other Names: Plastic scissor, Small Sharp/Sharp, Eye Suture Scissor

Similar Instruments with Same Inspections: Goldman Fox, Bonn, Knapp, LaGrange

Length: 3.5", 4" (curved), and 4.5" (straight)

    Most popular: 3.5" and 4" (curved)

Surgical Use: Very fine tissue dissection and cutting of fine suture

Tray Assembly Tips: Due to fragile nature of distal tips, the use of tip protectors is advised.

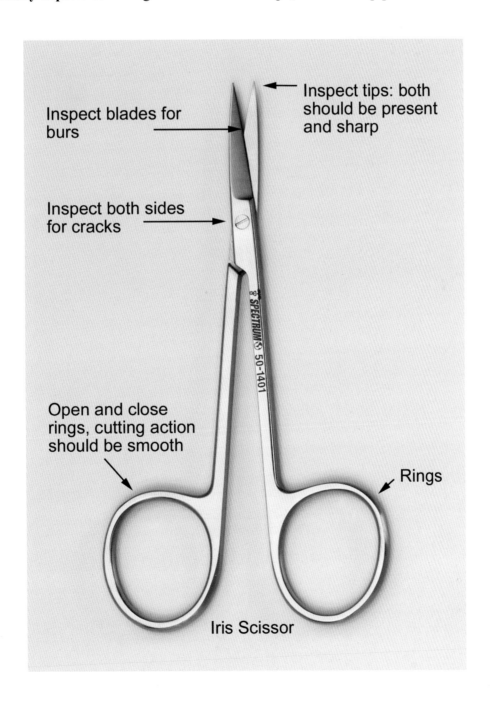

Inspect tips: both should be present and sharp

Inspect blades for burs

Inspect both sides for cracks

Open and close rings, cutting action should be smooth

Rings

Iris Scissor

Stevens Tenotomy Scissor

Proper Name: Stevens Tenotomy Scissor

Other Names: Tenotomy Scissor, Stevens Scissor

Similar Instruments With Same Inspection: Westcott Scissor

Blade Definition: Blades taper from mid-blade to the point. Sharp or blunt points

Length: 4" to 4.5"

Surgical Use: Ophthalmic, ENT, and plastic surgery tissue cutting

Sharpness Test Standard: Yellow scissor test material

Tray Assembly Tips: Keep rings slightly separated and tips of scissors going in same direction

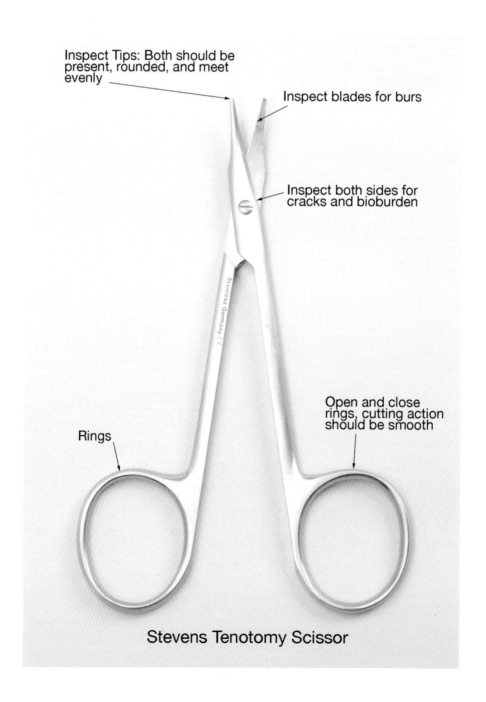

Inspect Tips: Both should be present, rounded, and meet evenly

Inspect blades for burs

Inspect both sides for cracks and bioburden

Open and close rings, cutting action should be smooth

Rings

Stevens Tenotomy Scissor

Strabismus Scissor

Proper Name: Strabismus Scissor

Other Names: Blunt Scissor

Similar Instruments With Same Inspection: Iris Scissor, Metzenbaum Scissor

Blade Definition: Small, rounded, blunt blades

Length: 4"

Surgical Use: Ophthalmic, ENT, and plastic surgery dissection scissor

Sharpness Test Standard: Yellow scissor test material

Tray Assembly Tips: Keep rings slightly separated and tips of scissors going in same direction

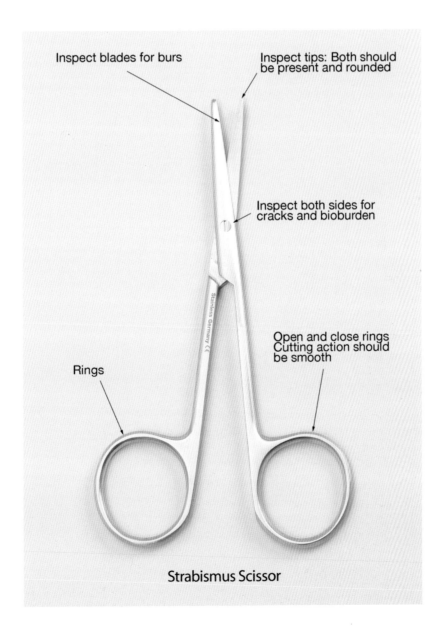

Inspect blades for burs

Inspect tips: Both should be present and rounded

Inspect both sides for cracks and bioburden

Open and close rings Cutting action should be smooth

Rings

Strabismus Scissor

Ribbon Iris

Proper Name: Ribbon Iris

Other Names: Big Ring Iris

Similar Instruments With Same Inspection: Any small dissection scissor

Blade Definition: Small pointed scissor blades

Length: 3.5", 4", 4.5"

Surgical Use: Fine dissection and cutting in plastic and ophthalmology surgery

Sharpness Test Standard: Yellow test material

Tray Assembly Tips: Keep rings slightly separated and tips of scissors going in same direction

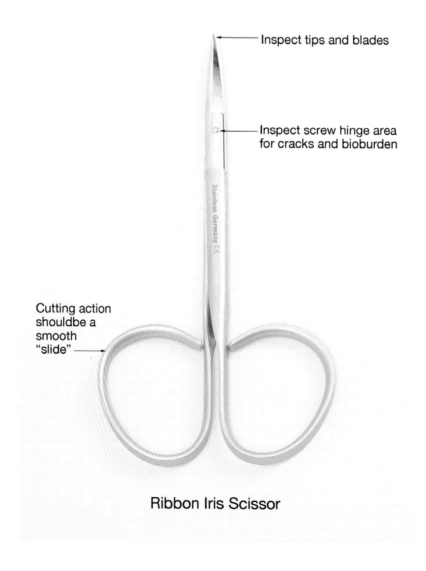

Inspect tips and blades

Inspect screw hinge area
for cracks and bioburden

Cutting action
shouldbe a
smooth
"slide"

Ribbon Iris Scissor

Ribbon Tenotomy

Proper Name: Ribbon Tenotomy

Other Names: Big Ring Tenotomy

Similar Instruments With Same Inspection: Any other small dissection scissor

Blade Definition: Semi-pointed blades

Length: 3.5", 4", 4.5"

Surgical Use: Fine tissue dissection and cutting in plastic and ophthalmology surgery

Sharpness Test Standard: Yellow test material

Tray Assembly Tips: Keep rings slightly separated and tips of scissors going in same direction

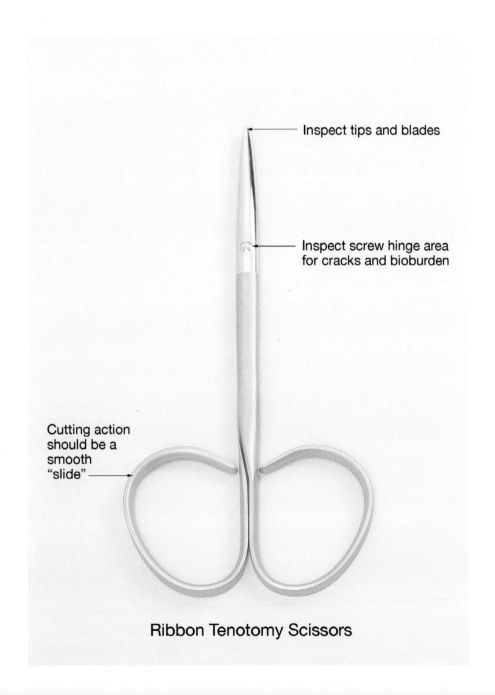

Inspect tips and blades

Inspect screw hinge area for cracks and bioburden

Cutting action should be a smooth "slide"

Ribbon Tenotomy Scissors

Jameson Strabismus Hook

Proper Name: Jameson Strabismus Hook

Similar Instruments: McGannon, Stevens, Green, VonGraefe Hook

Length: 5"

Tip/Blade Definition: Bulbous tip

Points of Inspection:

- Inspect edges for burs
- Inspect angle for 90°
- Inspect shaft

Surgical Use: Retraction of eye muscles

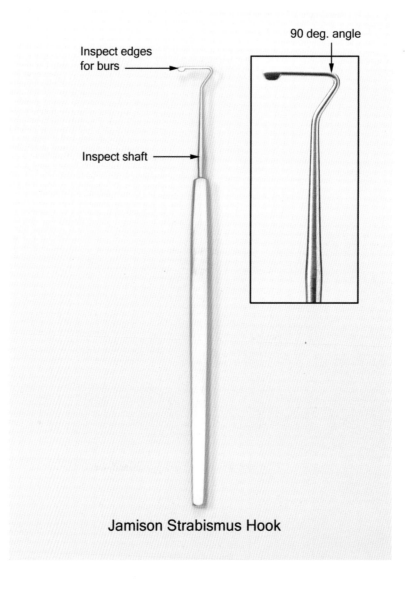

Jamison Strabismus Hook

Castroviejo Eye Speculum

Proper Name: Castroviejo Eye Speculum

Similar Instruments: Lancaster, Knapp, Lange, Williams, Guyton

Length: 3.75" and 4"

Tip definition: Fenestrated blades

Points of Inspection:

- Inspect blades for bioburden
- Inspect for cracks
- Test screw mechanism

Surgical Use: Hold eye lids open

Tray Assemble Tips: *DELICATE INSTRUMENT*; should be placed in a protective sterilization case with silicon mat.

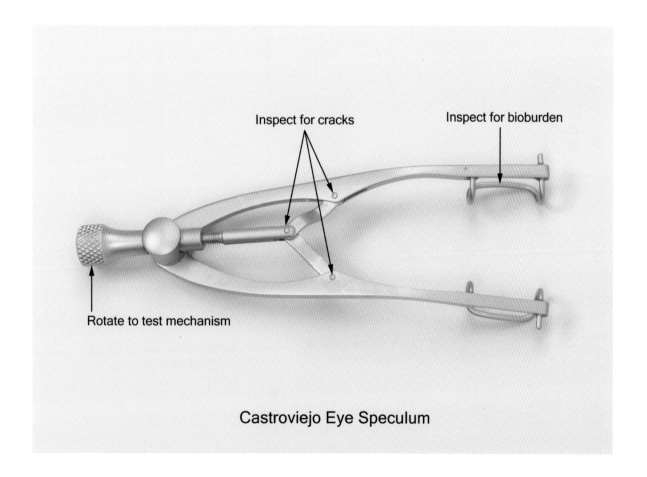

Castroviejo Eye Speculum

Eye Dressing Forcep

Proper Name: Eye Dressing Forcep

Similar Instruments: Iris Forcep, Oconnor

Length: 4"

Surgical Use: Fine tissue manipulation for ophthalmology procedure

Tray Assemble Tips: Instrument protection case is advised

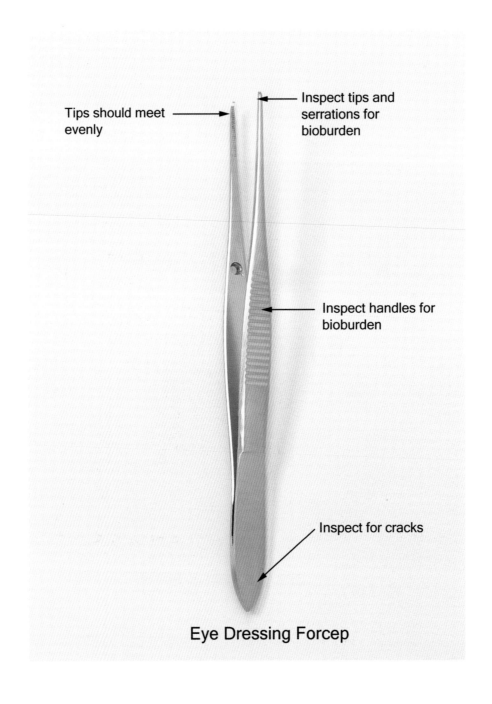

Tips should meet evenly

Inspect tips and serrations for bioburden

Inspect handles for bioburden

Inspect for cracks

Eye Dressing Forcep

Iris Tissue Forcep

Proper Name: Iris Tissue Forcep

Similar Instruments: Oconnor, Bracken, Foerster, Stevens

Length: 4"

Surgical Use: Fine tissue manipulation for ophthalmology procedures

Tray Assemble Tips: Instrument protection case advised

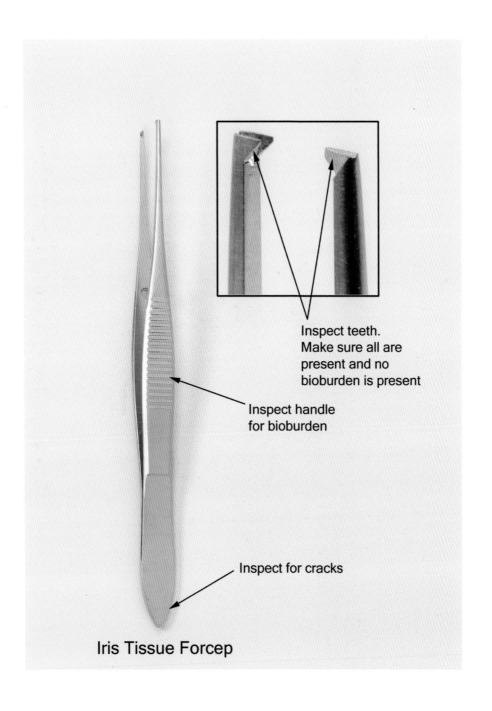

Inspect teeth.
Make sure all are
present and no
bioburden is present

Inspect handle
for bioburden

Inspect for cracks

Iris Tissue Forcep

Graefe Fixation Forcep

Proper Name: Graefe Fixation Forcep

Similar Instruments: Waldean, Guyton Noyes

Length: 4 3/8"

Tray Assemble Tips: Sterilize with lock in open position

Surgical Use: Manipulation of tissue

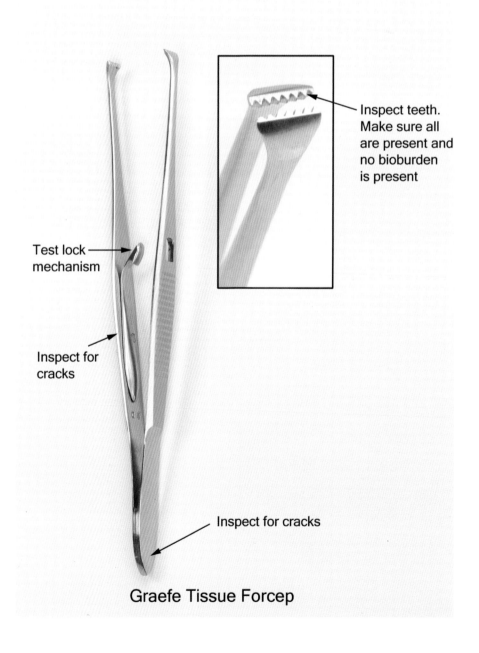

Inspect teeth.
Make sure all
are present and
no bioburden
is present

Test lock
mechanism

Inspect for
cracks

Inspect for cracks

Graefe Tissue Forcep

Castroviejo Suturing Forcep with Teeth

Proper Name: Castroviejo Suturing Forcep with teeth

Similar Instruments: Troutman, Barraquer, Pierse, Sauer

Length: 4"

Tray Assemble Tips: Instrument protection case is advised

Surgical Use: Manipulation and suturing assistance

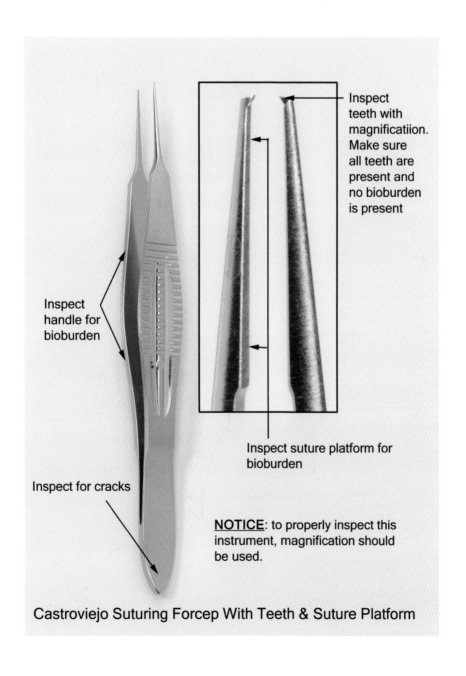

Inspect teeth with magnificatiion. Make sure all teeth are present and no bioburden is present

Inspect handle for bioburden

Inspect suture platform for bioburden

Inspect for cracks

<u>NOTICE</u>: to properly inspect this instrument, magnification should be used.

Castroviejo Suturing Forcep With Teeth & Suture Platform

Castroviejo Corneal Scissor

Proper Name: Castroviejo Corneal Scissor

Similar Instruments: Noyes, Barraquer, Westcott, McClure

Length: 4"

Tray Assemble Tips: Instrument protection case is advised

Surgical Use: Dissecting and cutting corneal tissue

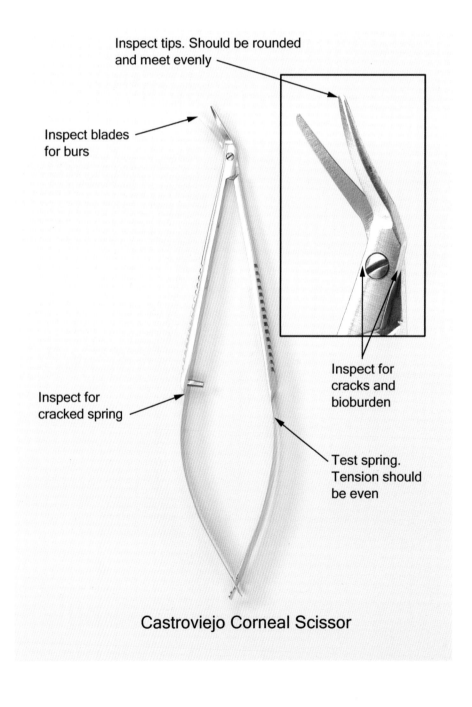

Castroviejo Corneal Scissor

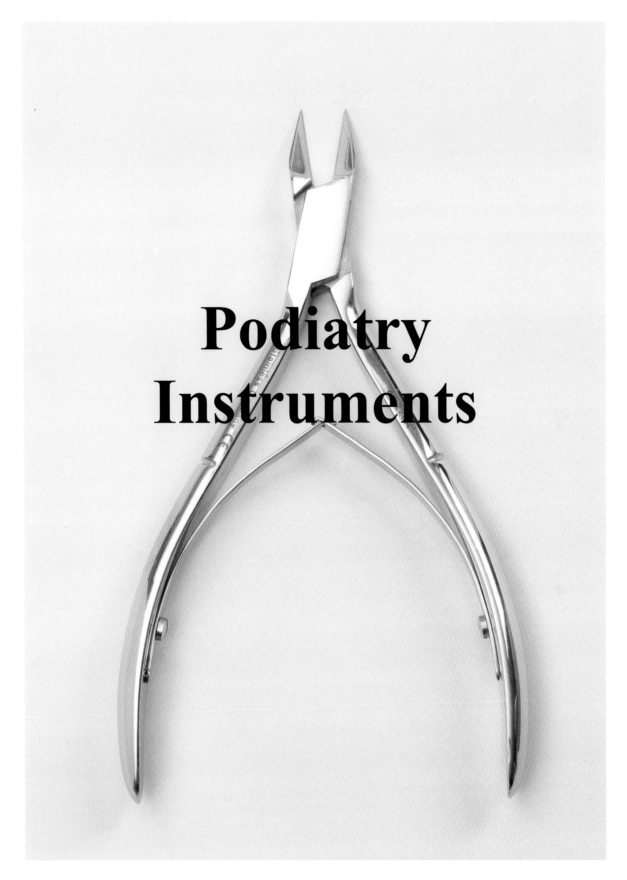

Podiatry
Instruments

Podiatry Instruments – used to treat diseases and disorders of the feet.

Nail Splitter

Proper Name: Nail Splitter

Other Names: English Anvil

Similar Instruments With Same Inspection: Nail Nippers, Nail Anvils

Blade Definition: Very pointed, flat blades

Length: 5" and 6"

Surgical Use: Splitting nail to trim for relief of pressure

Sharpness Test Standard: Index Card

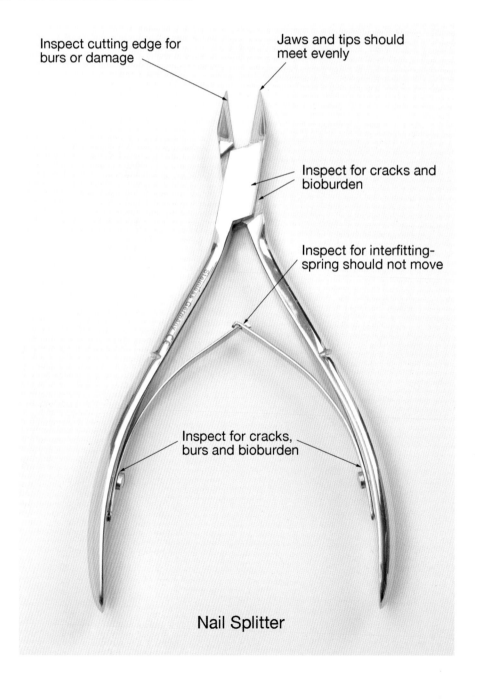

Inspect cutting edge for burs or damage

Jaws and tips should meet evenly

Inspect for cracks and bioburden

Inspect for interfitting-spring should not move

Inspect for cracks, burs and bioburden

Nail Splitter

Nail Nipper

Proper Name: Nail Nipper

Other Names: Nail Trimmers

Similar Instruments With Same Inspection: Nail Splitters

Blade Definition: Straight, sharp, pointed blades

Length: 4", 4.5", 5", 5.5", and 6"

Surgical Use: Trimming and/or removing finger or toenails

Sharpness Test Standard: Index Card

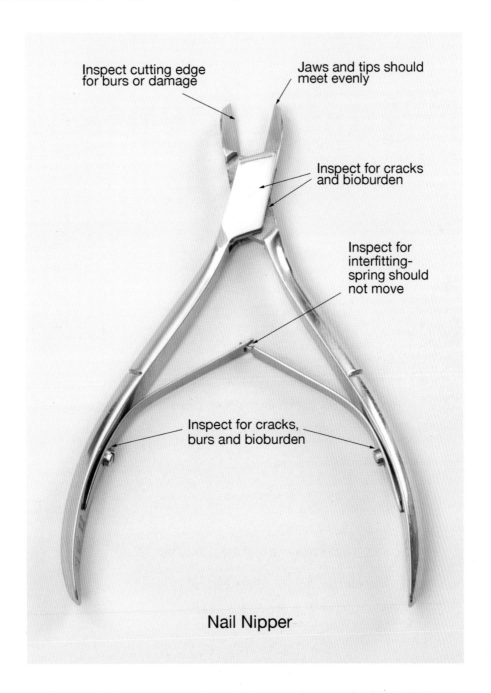

Inspect cutting edge for burs or damage

Jaws and tips should meet evenly

Inspect for cracks and bioburden

Inspect for interfitting- spring should not move

Inspect for cracks, burs and bioburden

Nail Nipper

Laparoscopic

Instruments

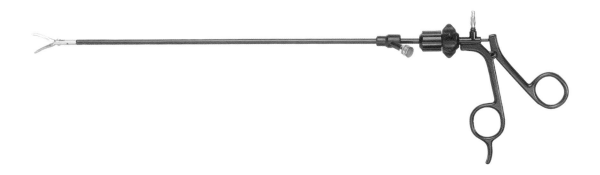

Laparoscopic Instruments – used to perform non-invasive surgical procedures, which increases the rate of recovery for the patient.

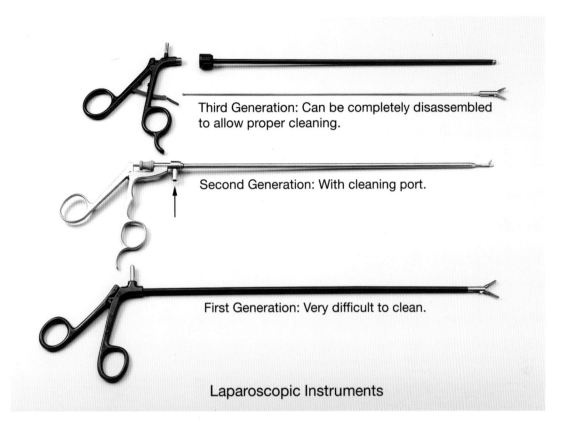

Third Generation: Can be completely disassembled to allow proper cleaning.

Second Generation: With cleaning port.

First Generation: Very difficult to clean.

Laparoscopic Instruments

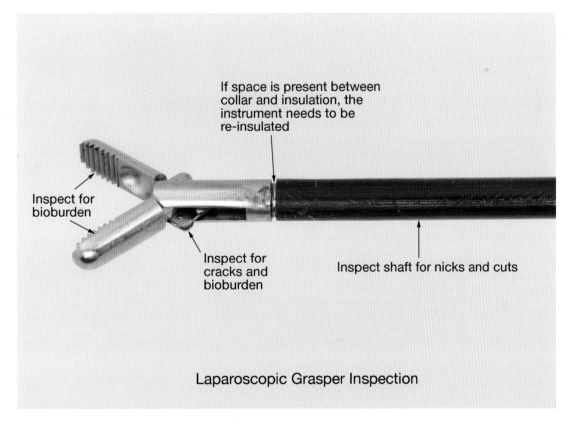

If space is present between collar and insulation, the instrument needs to be re-insulated

Inspect for bioburden

Inspect for cracks and bioburden

Inspect shaft for nicks and cuts

Laparoscopic Grasper Inspection

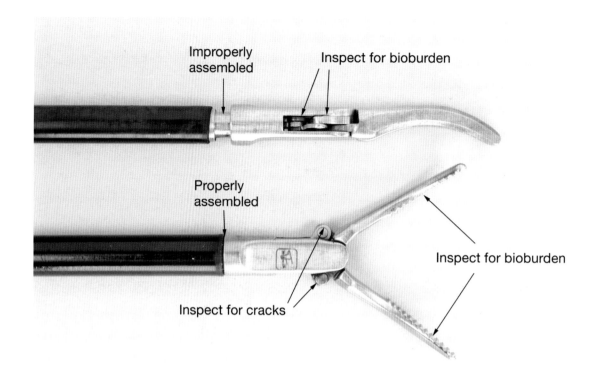

Improperly
assembled

Inspect for bioburden

Properly
assembled

Inspect for bioburden

Inspect for cracks

Grasper Inspection

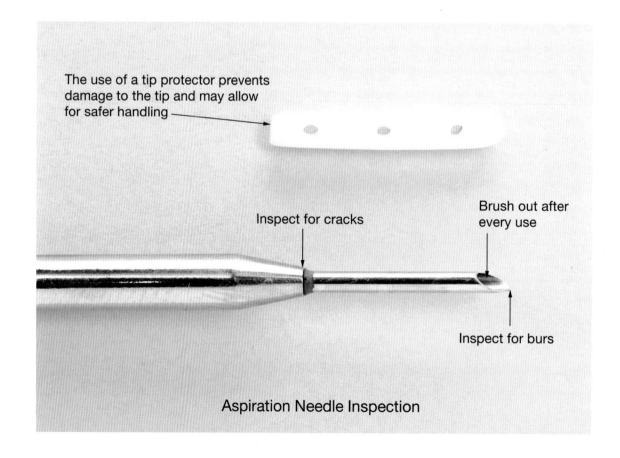

The use of a tip protector prevents
damage to the tip and may allow
for safer handling

Inspect for cracks

Brush out after
every use

Inspect for burs

Aspiration Needle Inspection

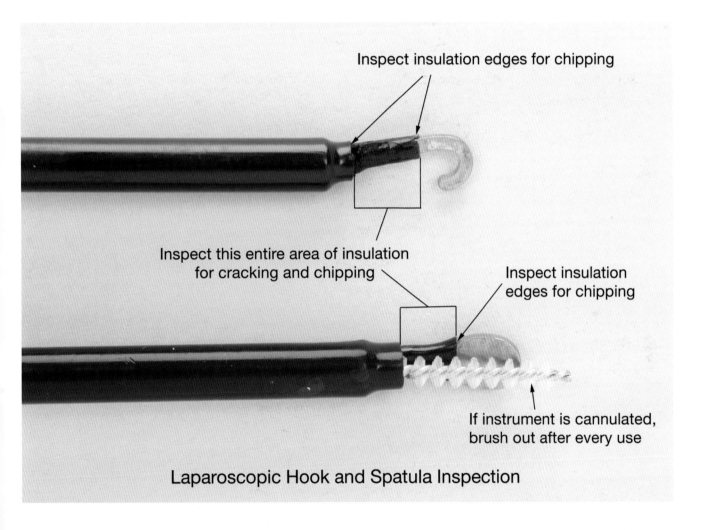

Inspect insulation edges for chipping

Inspect this entire area of insulation
for cracking and chipping

Inspect insulation
edges for chipping

If instrument is cannulated,
brush out after every use

Laparoscopic Hook and Spatula Inspection

Laparoscopic Insulation Testing

To test the insulation visually, inspect the entire shaft for any nicks or cuts. Next, lightly pull back on the insulation. If the insulation slides back, the instrument is in need of re-insulation.

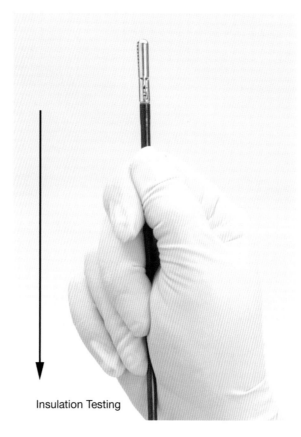

Insulation Testing

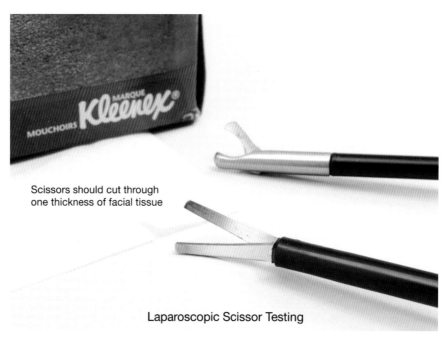

Scissors should cut through one thickness of facial tissue

Laparoscopic Scissor Testing

Sharpening Reusable Trocars

It is advisable to send the sheath out with the trocar when having the trocar sharpened. Having the two pieces (trocar with sheath) together, the repair company can evaluate if the facet goes under the distal end of the sheath. When this occurs, the trocar needs to be replaced.

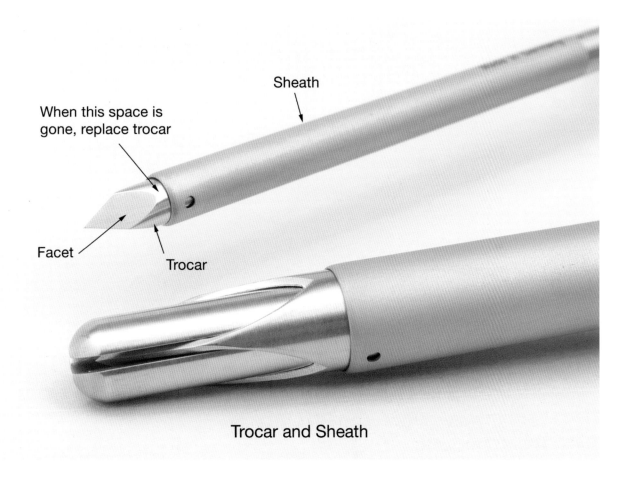

Trocar and Sheath

Evaluation of Linkage Wear

This test will determine if the inner linkage is worn, stretched, or fatigued. Wiggle the drive ring back and forth. If the jaw does not move, the linkage has been altered. This test also evaluates the surgeon's touch through the instrument. If the ring moves, the jaw should move as well.

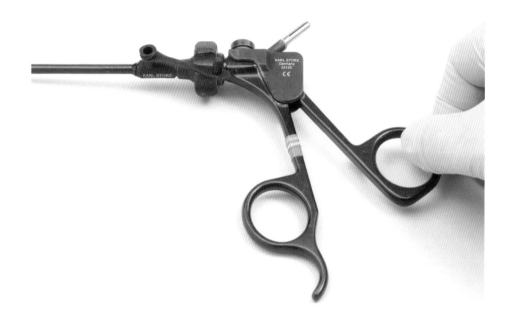

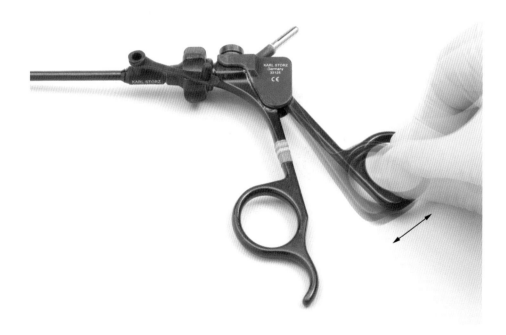

Proper Flushing and Irrigation

With distal tip underwater, connect syringe to irrigation port and draw up water from cleaning sink. Force cleaning fluids in and out of shaft.

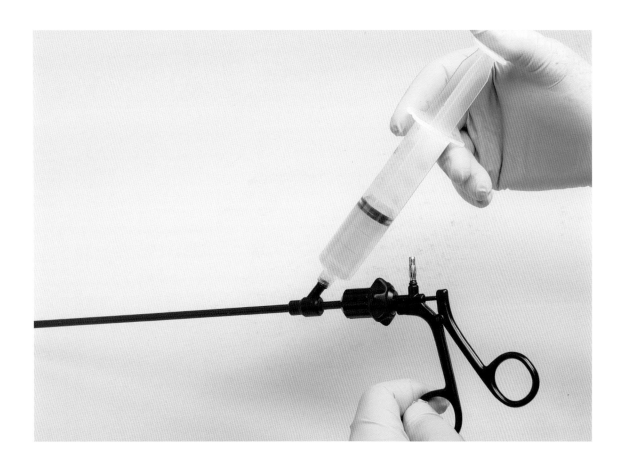

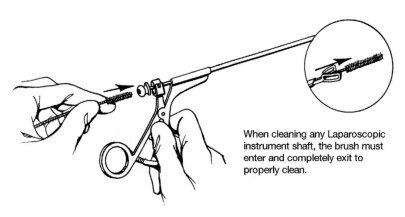

When cleaning any Laparoscopic instrument shaft, the brush must enter and completely exit to properly clean.

Vertical Soaking

When soaking Laparoscopic Instruments, soaking the instruments vertically allows fluid to enter at the distal tip and rise up. Fluids will seek their own level and this, in conjunction with an enzymatic cleaner, will assist with the cleaning process.

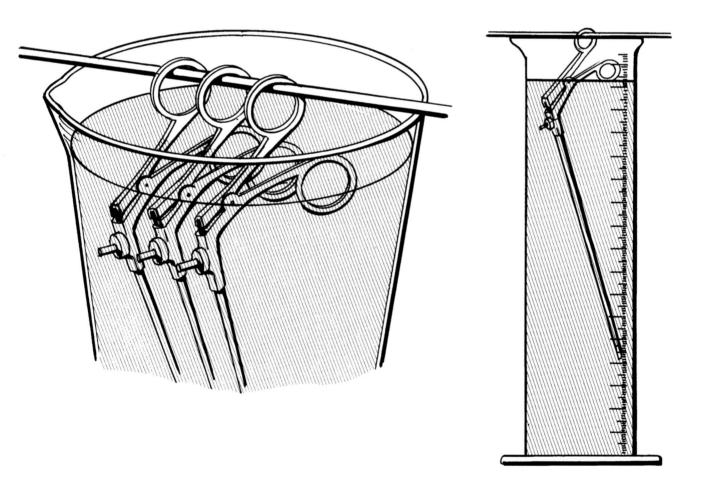

Index

Index

Index

Index

Index

Index

Index

Index

Index

Index

Index